Atlas of Cornea

Bharat Gurnani • Kirandeep Kaur
Editors

Atlas of Cornea

Springer

Editors
Bharat Gurnani
Department of Cataract, Cornea,
Trauma, External Diseases, Ocular
Surface and Refractive Services
Gomabai Netralaya and Research Centre
Neemuch, Madhya Pradesh, India

Kirandeep Kaur
Department of Cataract, Pediatric
Ophthalmology and Strabismus
Gomabai Netralaya and Research Centre
Neemuch, Madhya Pradesh, India

ISBN 978-981-96-0012-0 ISBN 978-981-96-0013-7 (eBook)
https://doi.org/10.1007/978-981-96-0013-7

This Springer imprint is published by the registered company Springer Nature Singapore Pte Ltd.
The registered company address is: 152 Beach Road, #21-01/04 Gateway East, Singapore 189721, Singapore

Contents

Ocular Surface Disease

1

Shweta Agarwal, Bhaskar Srinivasan, Geetha Iyer,
Bharat Gurnani, and Kirandeep Kaur

1.1 Introduction

Ocular surface disease encompasses a wide range of disorders that affect the surface of the eye, including the tear film, conjunctiva, and cornea. These conditions can significantly impact a patient's quality of life, causing discomfort, visual disturbance, and sometimes leading to more severe complications. This chapter provides an overview of various ocular surface diseases, including dry eye, rosacea, seborrheic blepharitis, staphylococcal blepharitis, staphylococcal blepharoconjunctivitis, marginal keratitis, phlyctenular keratoconjunctivitis (phlyctenulosis), hordeola, and chalazia. Understanding and managing ocular surface diseases require a comprehensive approach that includes accurate diagnosis, appropriate treatment, and patient education. This chapter provides an in-depth exploration of these conditions, highlighting the importance of tailored therapeutic strategies to improve patient outcomes and enhance their quality of life. Through a combination of medical, surgical, and supportive interventions, effective management of ocular surface diseases can be achieved, ensuring better ocular health and overall well-being for affected individuals.

1.2 Various Manifestations of Dry Eyes

1.2.1 Punctate Epithelial Erosions

Dry eye disease (DED) is one of the most common ocular surface disorders, characterized by a deficiency in the quantity or quality of tears, leading to ocular discomfort and visual disturbance. It can result from various factors, including aging, hormonal changes, autoimmune diseases, and environmental conditions. The mainstay of treatment involves artificial tears, anti-inflammatory medications, and lifestyle modifications to alleviate symptoms and improve tear film stability [1].

S. Agarwal (✉) · B. Srinivasan · G. Iyer
CJ Shah Cornea Services, Medical Research Foundation, Sankara Nethralaya, Chennai, Tamil Nadu, India

B. Gurnani
Department of Cataract, Cornea, Trauma, External Diseases, Ocular Surface and Refractive Services, Gomabai Netralaya and Research Centre, Neemuch, Madhya Pradesh, India

K. Kaur
Department of Cataract, Pediatric Ophthalmology and Strabismus, Gomabai Netralaya and Research Centre, Neemuch, Madhya Pradesh, India

B. Gurnani, K. Kaur (eds.), *Atlas of Cornea*, https://doi.org/10.1007/978-981-96-0013-7_1

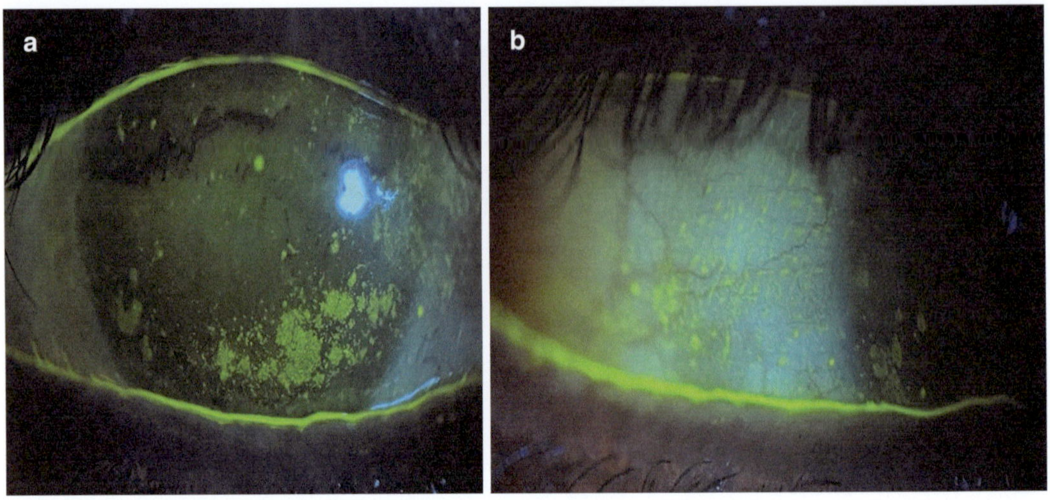

Diffuse illumination slit lamp image of a patient depicting (**a**) corneal staining in the form of punctate epithelial erosions and (**b**) conjunctival staining in dry eye disease

1.2.2 Filamentary Keratitis

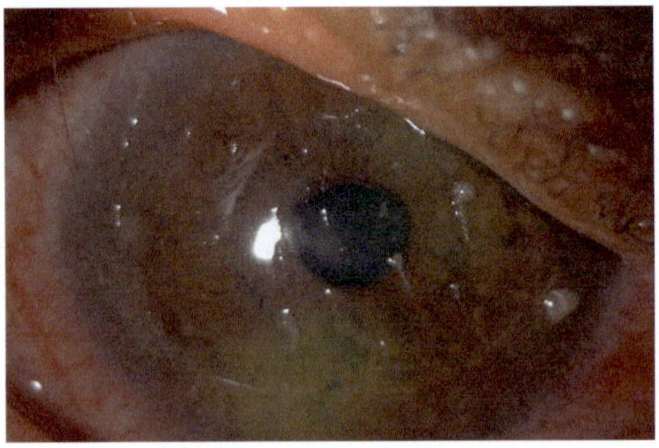

Diffuse illumination slit lamp image of a patient with severe dry eye disease depicting filaments and inferior quadrant corneal staining

1.2.3 Sterile Corneal Melt

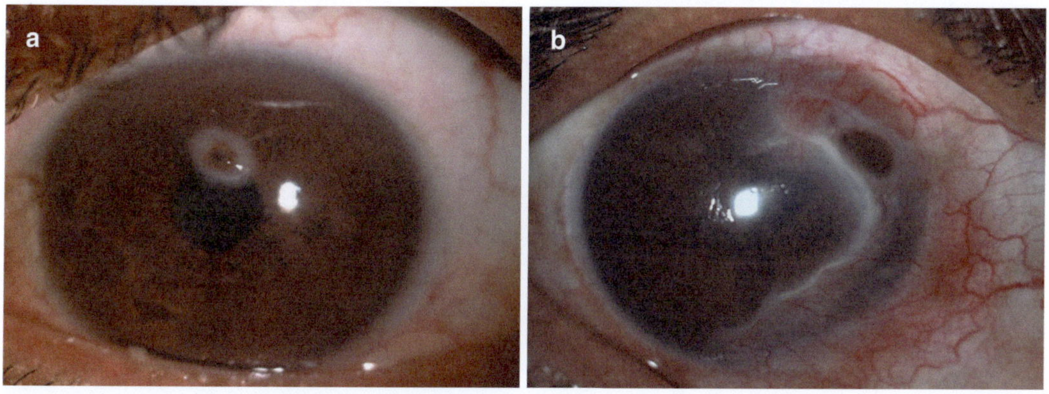

(**a**) Diffuse illumination slit lamp image of a patient depicting sterile melt with iris prolapse in a case of uncontrolled rheumatoid arthritis with severe dry eye; (**b**) Diffuse illumination slit lamp image of another patient depicting conjunctival inflammation and descemetocele in a case of peripheral ulcerative keratitis

1.2.4 Inflammatory Dry Eyes

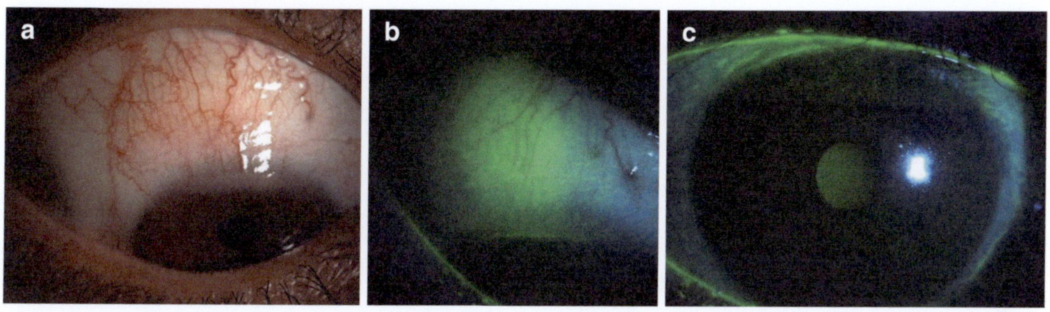

Diffuse illumination slit lamp image of a patient with inflammatory dry eyes depicting. (**a**) Hyperemic superior bulbar conjunctiva indicating inflammation. (**b**, **c**) Corresponding increased staining of the conjunctiva and superior cornea appreciated in yellow filter

1.2.5 Severe Inflammation with Limbal Stem Cell Deficiency

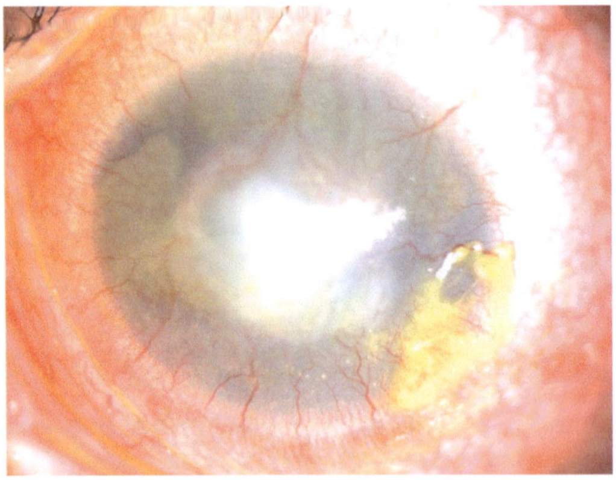

Diffuse illumination slit lamp image of a patient with inflammatory dry eyes depicting diffuse conjunctival congestion, 360 degree limbal stem cell deficiency, corneal neovascularization, central leukomatous corneal scarring, and lipid keratopathy from 3 to 4 o' clock quadrant

1.2.6 Conjunctival and Corneal Staining

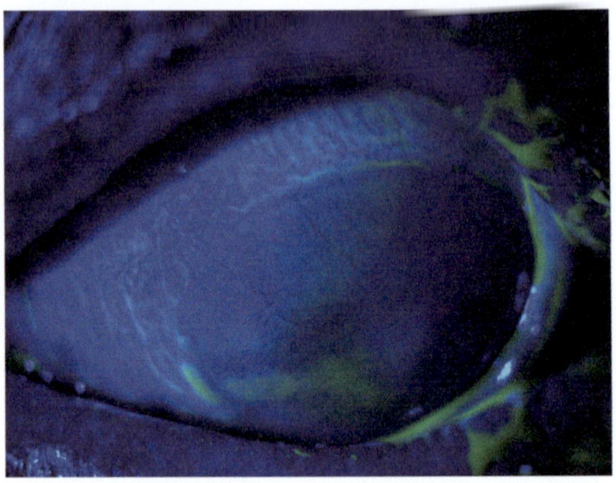

Diffuse illumination cobalt blue filter image of a patient with severe dry eyes depicting corneal and conjunctival staining in all quadrants

1.2.7 Lid Wiper Epitheliopathy

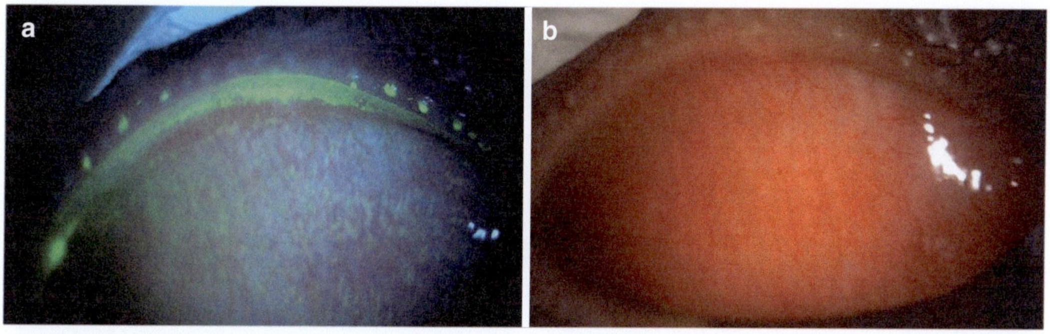

Diffuse illumination slit lamp image of a patient with dry eyes depicting: (**a**) Linear staining in the lid wiper area between the posterior lid margin and the subtarsal fold extending along the entire length of the lid indicating severe lid wiper epitheliopathy and (**b**) Significant hyperemia of the lid wiper area along with the upper tarsal conjunctiva

1.2.8 Lid Wiper Epitheliopathy

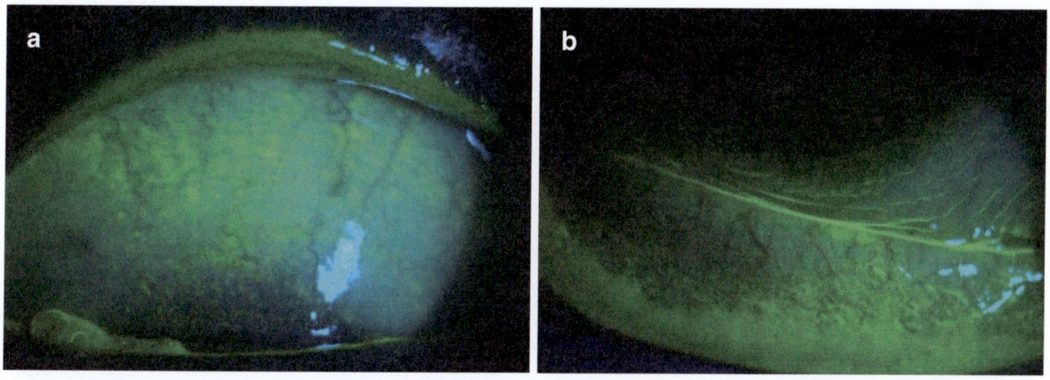

Slit lamp image of a patient with dry eye disease depicting linear staining in the lid wiper area between the posterior lid margin and the subtarsal fold extending along the entire length of the lid indicating severe lid wiper epitheliopathy both in the upper (**a**) and lower (**b**) lids

1.2.9 Neurotrophic Dry Eyes

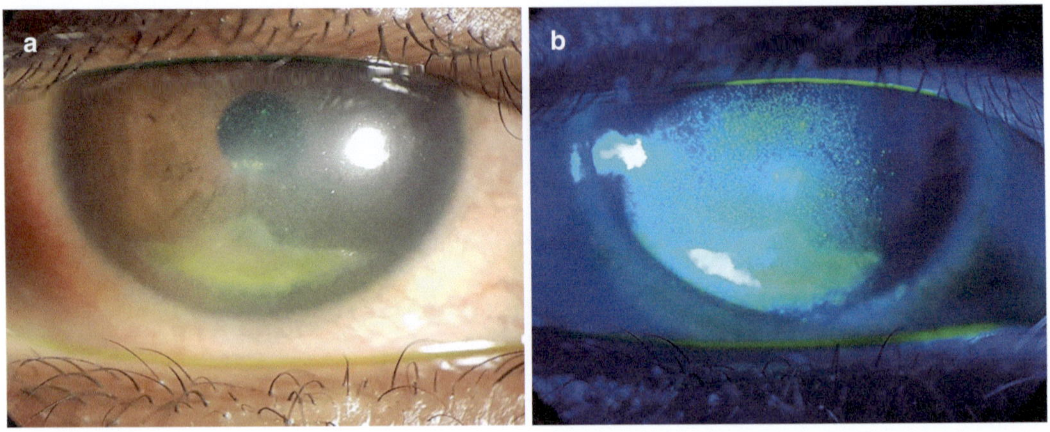

Diffuse illumination slit lamp image of a patient with neurotrophic keratopathy depicting. (**a**) Corneal staining in the inferior quadrant with exposure keratopathy. (**b**) Cobalt blue filter picture of the same patient depicting diffuse punctate epithelial erosions and exposure of keratopathy in the inferior quadrant

1.2.10 Pre- and Postpunctal Cautery

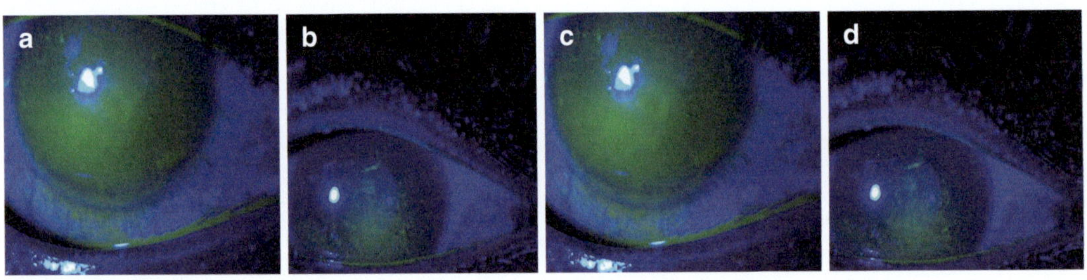

Diffuse illumination cobalt blue filter slit lamp image of the patient depicting: (**a**, **b**) Diffuse SPKs in severe dry eye prepunctal cautery; (**c**, **d**) 2 weeks following punctal cautery, almost complete resolution of SPKs noted

1.2.11 Neurotrophic Keratitis

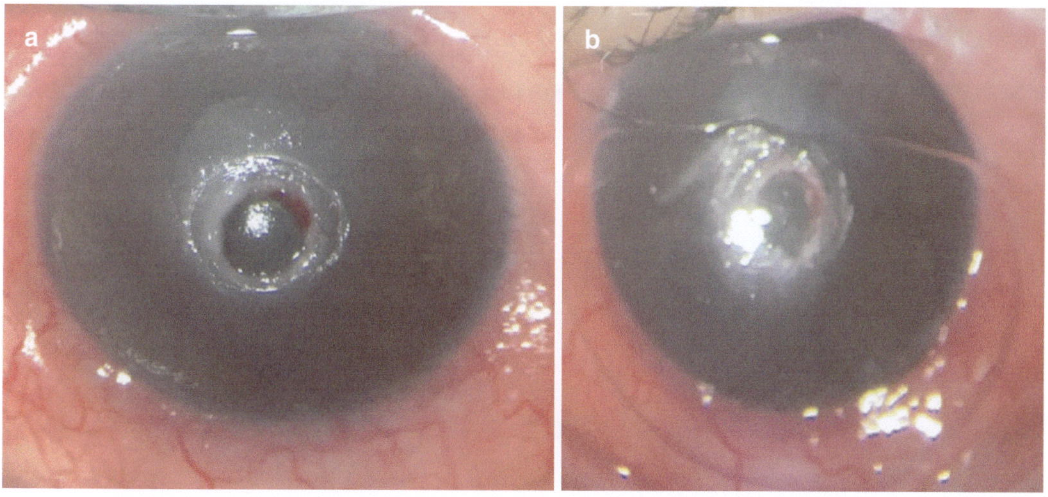

Diffuse illumination slit lamp image of a patient depicting: (**a**) Central punched out area of thinning in a neurotrophic cornea. (**b**) Cyanoacrylate glue applied to prevent perforation along with bandage contact lens

1.2.12 Recurrent Chalazion

Chalazia are chronic, sterile granulomatous inflammations of the meibomian glands, often resulting from unresolved hordeola. They present as painless nodules on the eyelid. Management includes warm compresses, lid massage, and in persistent cases, surgical incision and curettage [2].

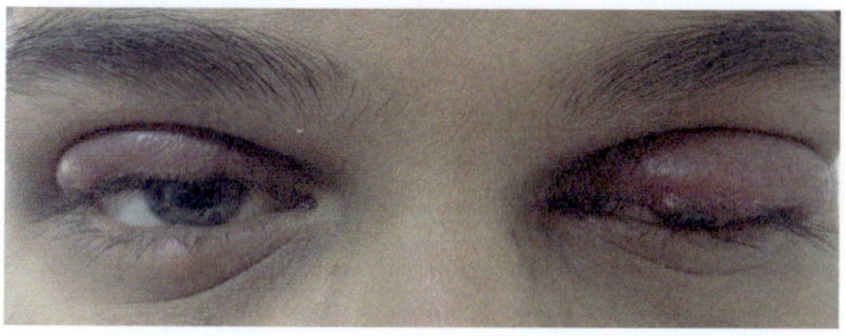

Diffuse illumination gross image of a patient depicting recurrent chalazia in an otherwise healthy 16-year-old child

1.2.13 Staphylococcal Marginal Keratitis

Marginal keratitis is an inflammatory condition affecting the peripheral cornea, often associated with blepharitis. It is characterized by small, peripheral corneal infiltrates that cause discomfort and photophobia. Management typically involves the use of topical steroids and antibiotics to reduce inflammation and prevent infection [3].

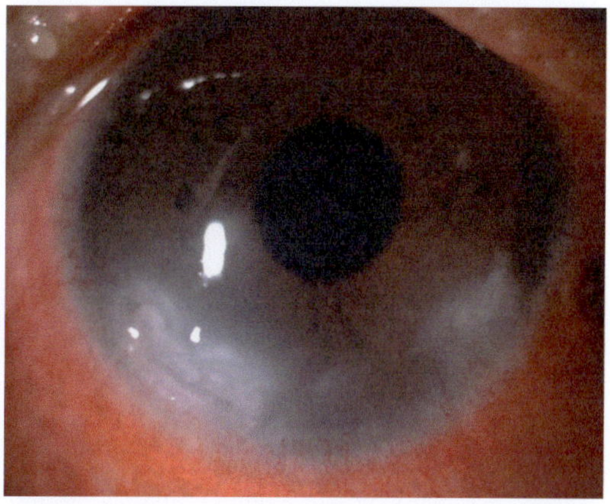

Diffuse illumination slit lamp image of a patient depicting marginal keratitis in a patient with capped meibomian orifices

1.3 Meibomian Gland Disease

1.3.1 Obstructive Meibomian Glands with Telangiectasia

Meibomian gland disease (MGD) is a chronic condition characterized by the dysfunction of the meibomian glands, leading to altered lipid composition of the tear film and evaporative dry eye. Management includes warm compresses, lid hygiene, oral tetracyclines, and other treatments to improve gland function and tear film stability [4].

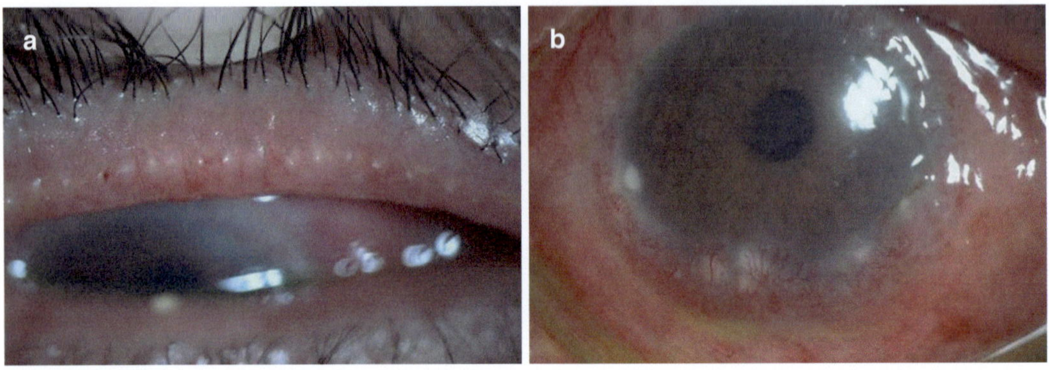

Diffuse illumination slit lamp image of a patient depicting: (**a**) Thick inflamed lid margin with telangiectasia and blocked meibomian orifices. (**b**) Sterile immune infiltrates in the peripheral cornea indicating marginal keratitis along with an inflamed surface

1.3.2 Epidermolysis Bullosa

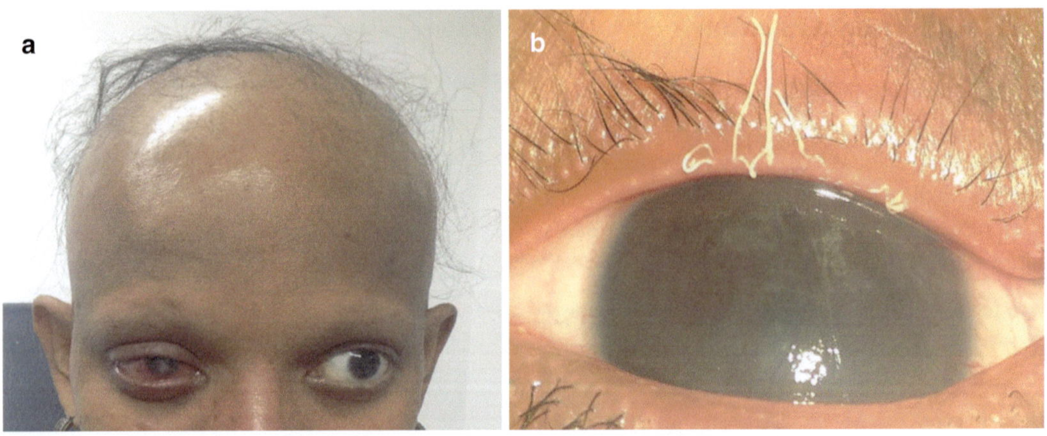

(**a**) Gross image of a patient depicting loss of hair and eyelashes in a child with epidermolysis bullosa presenting with recurrent redness and photophobia. (**b**) Diffuse illumination slit lamp image of a patient depicting thick cheesy secretions from blocked meibomian orifices in a child with epidermolysis bullosa

1.3.3 Demodex Blepharitis

Demodex blepharitis is caused by an infestation of Demodex mites on the eyelashes and eyelids. It presents with symptoms of itching, burning, and foreign body sensation. Treatment involves eyelid hygiene, tea tree oil, and other acaricidal treatments to reduce mite infestation and alleviate symptoms [5].

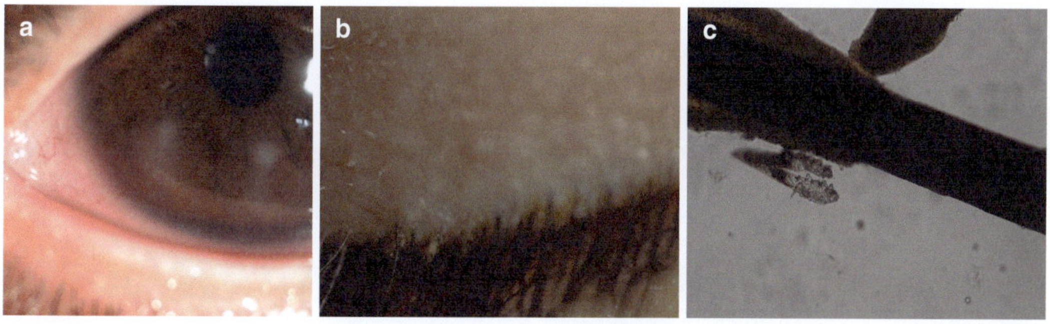

(**a**) Diffuse illumination slit lamp image of a patient depicting whitish immune infiltrates seen in the inferior half of the cornea with superficial corneal vascularization. (**b**) Gross illumination image of a patient depicting cylindrical dandruff around eyelashes causing recurrent ocular surface inflammation, indicating Demodex blepharitis. (**c**) Demodex seen in the epilated eyelash under a microscope

1.3.4 Superior Limbic Keratoconjunctivitis (SLKC)

Superior limbic keratoconjunctivitis (SLK) is a chronic inflammatory condition affecting the superior conjunctiva and cornea. It is often associated with thyroid disease and presents with symptoms of redness, foreign body sensation, and photophobia. Treatment includes topical steroids, lubricants, and in some cases, surgical intervention to alleviate symptoms and prevent recurrence [6].

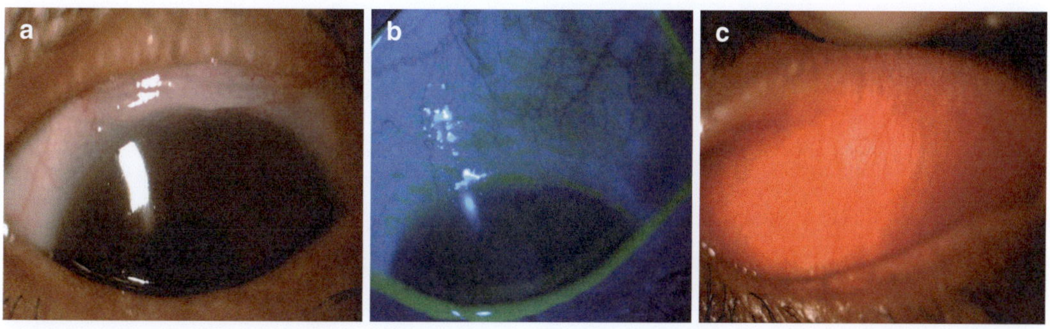

(**a**) Diffuse illumination slit lamp image of a patient depicting superior redundant conjunctiva that can be identified by a slight push of the upper lid on the bulbar surface. (**b**) Diffuse illumination cobalt blue image of a patient depicting fluorescein staining of the superior conjunctiva. (**c**) Diffuse illumination slit lamp image of the corresponding papillary reaction in the upper tarsal surface due to friction

1.4 Phlyctenulosis

1.4.1 Conjunctivitis: Staining under Cobalt Blue Filter

Phlyctenular keratoconjunctivitis is an immune-mediated response to bacterial antigens, often associated with staphylococcal blepharitis or tuberculosis. It presents as small, white nodules on the conjunctiva or cornea, accompanied by redness and tearing. Treatment includes addressing the underlying infection with antibiotics and reducing inflammation with steroids [7].

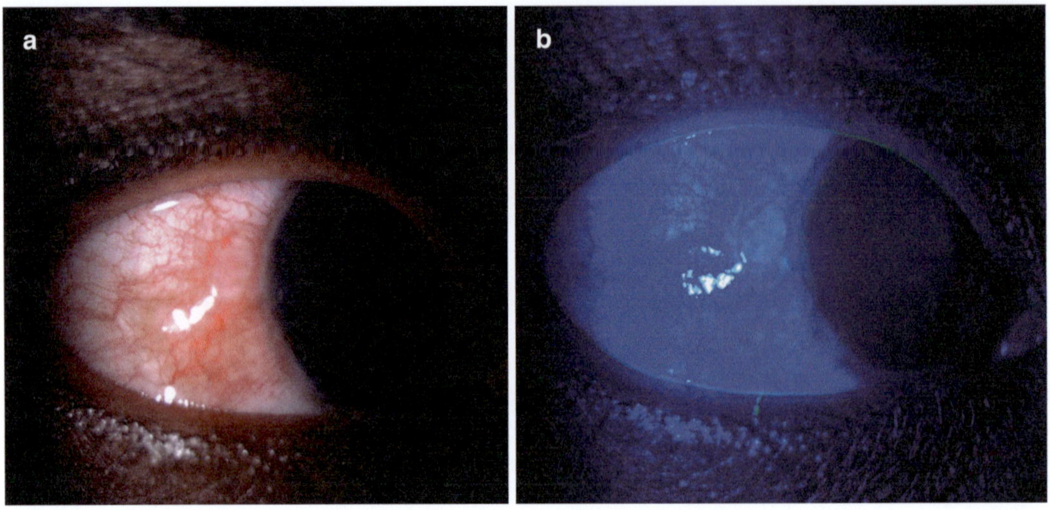

(**a**) Diffuse illumination slit lamp image of a patient depicting temporal conjunctival and episcleral congestion, elevated nodular growth abutting the limbus at 9 o' clock with surface ulceration suggestive of phlyctenular conjunctivitis. (**b**) Diffuse illumination cobalt blue image of the same patient depicting staining of the conjunctival ulcer

1.4.2 Conjunctivitis

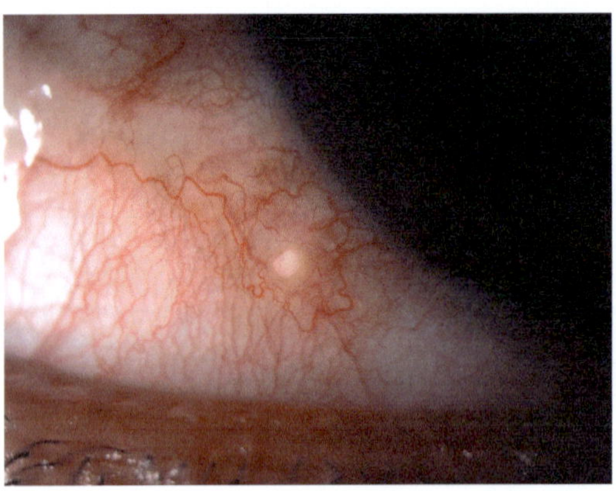

Diffuse illumination slit lamp image of a patient depicting temporal conjunctival and episcleral congestion, small elevated nodular growth with surface ulceration suggestive of phlyctenular conjunctivitis

1.5 Rosacea

1.5.1 Blepharoconjunctivitis

Ocular rosacea is a manifestation of rosacea that affects the eyes, often leading to chronic inflammation of the eyelids, conjunctiva, and cornea. Symptoms include redness, burning, and irritation. Management includes eyelid hygiene, oral antibiotics like doxycycline, and topical treatments to control inflammation and prevent complications such as corneal damage [8].

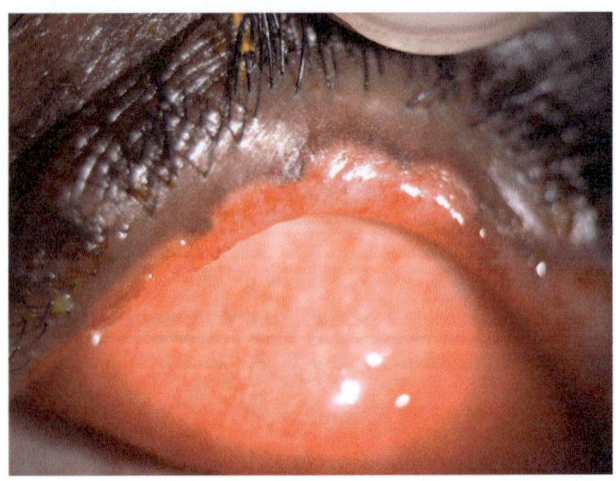

Diffuse illumination slit lamp image of a patient with rosacea ulcerative blepharitis depicting blepharitis with upper lid margin ulceration and inflammation along with upper tarsal conjunctival hyperemia

1.5.2 Lid Margin Ulceration

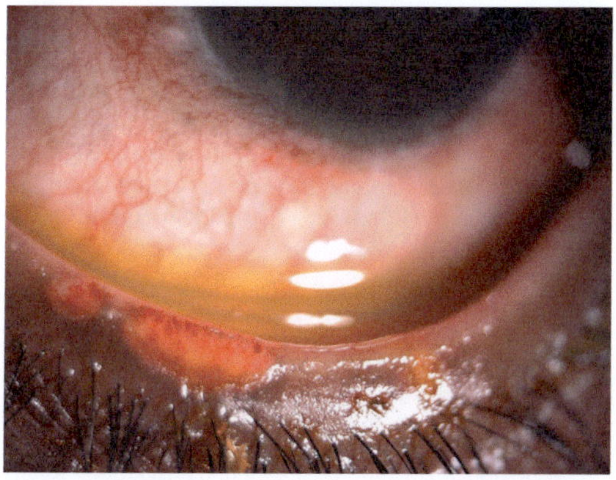

Diffuse illumination slit lamp image of a patient with rosacea ulcerative blepharitis depicting blepharitis with lower lid margin ulceration and inflammation along with upper tarsal conjunctival congestion and limbitis

1.5.3 Marginal Keratitis

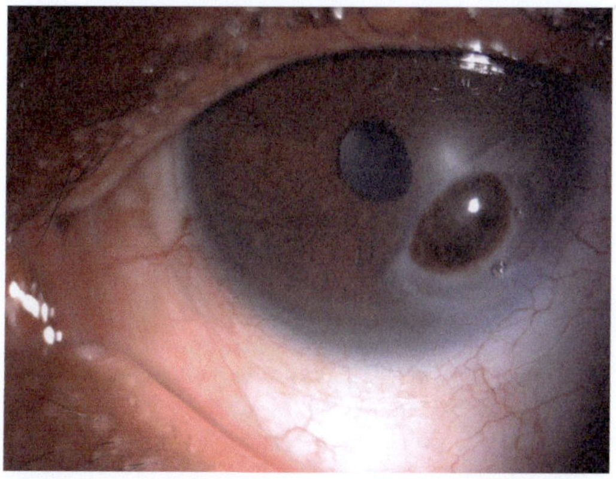

Diffuse illumination slit lamp image of a patient with rosacea, marginal keratitis, and blepharitis, depicting blepharitis, corneal thinning in the nasal quadrant along with descemetocele formation

1.5.4 Seborrheic Blepharitis

Seborrheic blepharitis is a chronic inflammatory condition affecting the eyelids, often associated with seborrheic dermatitis. It is characterized by redness, scaling, and dandruff-like flakes on the eyelashes. Treatment focuses on maintaining eyelid hygiene, using antidandruff shampoos, and occasionally topical steroids to reduce inflammation [9].

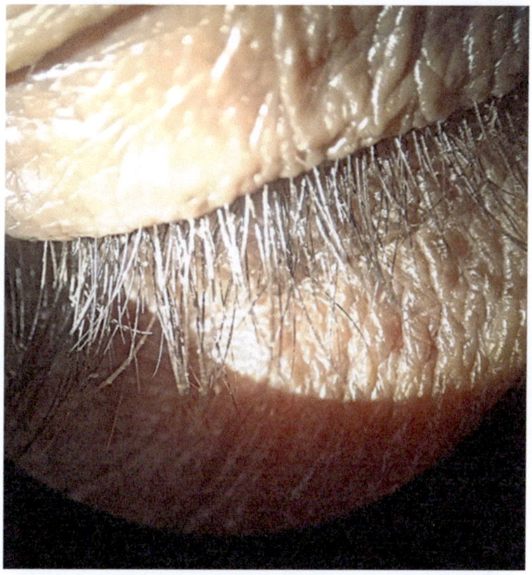

Digital image of a patient depicting diffuse seborrheic blepharitis in the upper eyelashes

1.5.5 Staphylococcal Blepharitis

Staphylococcal blepharitis is caused by bacterial infection of the eyelids, particularly by Staphylococcus species. It presents with symptoms of irritation, crusting, and eyelid redness. Management includes eyelid hygiene, antibiotic ointments, and in some cases, oral antibiotics to control the bacterial load and alleviate symptoms [10].

1.6 Staphylococcal Blepharoconjunctivitis

This condition is a combination of staphylococcal blepharitis and conjunctivitis, where the infection extends to the conjunctiva. Symptoms include redness, discharge, and discomfort. Treatment involves a combination of antibiotic eye drops and ointments, along with rigorous eyelid hygiene practices [10].

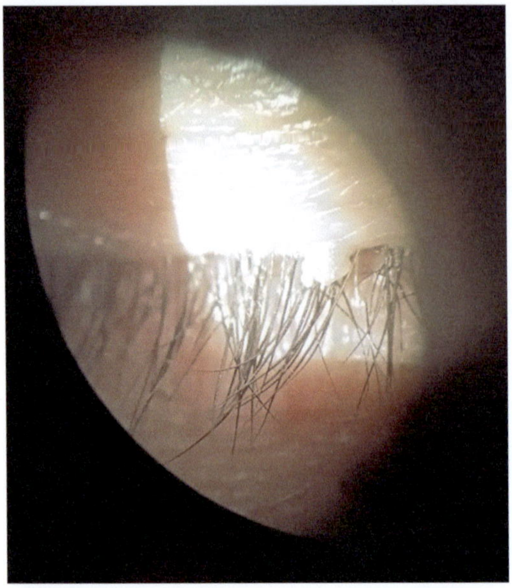

Digital image of a patient depicting staphylococcal blepharitis with crusting and scaling

1.6.1 Hordeola

Hordeola, commonly known as styes, are acute infections of the eyelid glands, typically caused by *Staphylococcus aureus*. They present as painful, red swellings on the eyelid margin. Treatment includes warm compresses to promote drainage, and antibiotics if there is an associated infection [11].

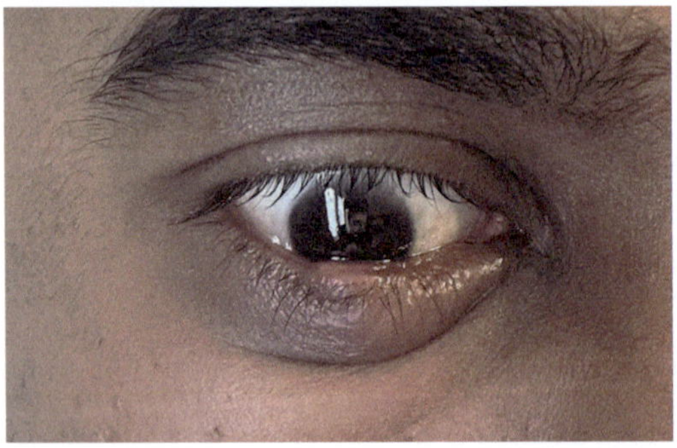

Digital gross image of a patient depicting lower lid hordeolum externum

References

1. Craig JP, Nelson JD, Azar DT, Belmonte C, Bron AJ, Chauhan SK, et al. TFOS DEWS II report. Ocul Surf. 2017;15(3):276–83. https://doi.org/10.1016/j.jtos.2017.05.006.
2. Goawalla A, Lee V. A prospective study of intralesional triamcinolone for primary and recurrent chalazia. Eye (Lond). 2017;31(6):894–9. https://doi.org/10.1038/eye.2016.270.
3. Dharamsothi PR, Smith AF, Liu C, Toma HS, Tuli SS. Management of marginal keratitis. Surv Ophthalmol. 2016;61(6):689–93. https://doi.org/10.1016/j.survophthal.2016.01.004.
4. Geerling G, Tauber J, Baudouin C, Goto E, Matsumoto Y, O'Brien T, et al. The international workshop on Meibomian gland dysfunction: report of the subcommittee on management and treatment of Meibomian gland dysfunction. Invest Ophthalmol Vis Sci. 2011;52(4):2050–64.
5. Liu J, Sheha H, Tseng SC. Pathogenic role of Demodex mites in blepharitis. Curr Opin Allergy Clin Immunol. 2010;10(5):505–10.
6. Kinoshita S, Yokoi N, Sugita J, Saito I, Sotozono C. Superior limbic keratoconjunctivitis. Semin Ophthalmol. 1995;10(1):57–61.
7. Abdellah MM, Said DG, Dua HS. Management of phlyctenular keratoconjunctivitis. Surv Ophthalmol. 2015;60(1):1–14. https://doi.org/10.1016/j.survophthal.2014.05.002.
8. Vieira AC, Höfling-Lima AL, Mannis MJ. Ocular rosacea—a review. Arq Bras Oftalmol. 2017;80(3):202–6. https://doi.org/10.5935/0004-2749.20170050.
9. Foulks GN, Borchman D, Yappert M, Kakar S, Podoll N. Topical azithromycin and oral doxycycline therapy of meibomian gland dysfunction: a comparative clinical and spectroscopic pilot study. Cornea. 2016;35(4):500–6. https://doi.org/10.1097/ICO.0000000000000736.
10. Lindsley K, Matsumura S, Hatef E, Mckoy NA, Kuo IC. Interventions for chronic blepharitis. Cochrane Database Syst Rev. 2016;2016:2.
11. Mahaling B, Satyanarayan A. Clinical profile and treatment outcomes in patients with hordeolum externum. Int J Ophthalmol. 2018;11(6):1068–72. https://doi.org/10.18240/ijo.2018.06.22.

Eyelid, Conjunctival, and Corneal Conditions Associated with Ocular Surface Disorders

2

Prateek Tiwari, Bharat Gurnani, and Kirandeep Kaur

2.1 Introduction

Ocular surface disorders encompass a broad range of conditions affecting the eyelids, conjunctiva, and cornea, often leading to significant visual impairment and discomfort. These conditions are multifactorial in etiology, ranging from inflammatory, infectious, and degenerative to traumatic origins. Understanding these disorders is crucial for developing effective treatment strategies and improving patient outcomes. This introduction provides an overview of several key ocular surface disorders, including superior limbic keratoconjunctivitis (SLK), conjunctivochalasis, Stevens-Johnson syndrome (SJS), conjunctival disease and surface disorders of the cornea (including ocular surface squamous neoplasia [OSSN]), exposure keratopathy, neurotrophic keratopathy, recurrent corneal erosion, dellen, limbal stem cell deficiency, Tenon's patch graft, vernal keratoconjunctivitis, pterygium, meibomitis, pyogenic granuloma, band-shaped keratopathy, chemical injury, corneal scar, anterior staphyloma, auto-evisceration, corneal ulcer, and conjunctival granuloma.

2.2 Ocular Surface Squamous Neoplasia

2.2.1 Gelatinous OSSN

Ocular surface squamous neoplasia (OSSN) encompasses a spectrum from mild dysplasia to invasive squamous cell carcinoma of the conjunctiva and cornea. Risk factors include UV exposure, HPV infection, and immunosuppression. Diagnosis involves clinical examination and biopsy, with treatment options including surgical excision, cryotherapy, and topical chemotherapeutics such as mitomycin C and 5-fluorouracil [1].

P. Tiwari
Cornea and Refractive Services, Antardrashti Netralaya, Indore, Madhya Pradesh, India

B. Gurnani (✉)
Department of Cataract, Cornea, Trauma, External Diseases, Ocular Surface and Refractive Services, Gomabai Netralaya and Research Centre, Neemuch, Madhya Pradesh, India

K. Kaur
Department of Cataract, Pediatric Ophthalmology and Strabismus, Gomabai Netralaya and Research Centre, Neemuch, Madhya Pradesh, India

B. Gurnani, K. Kaur (eds.), *Atlas of Cornea*, https://doi.org/10.1007/978-981-96-0013-7_2

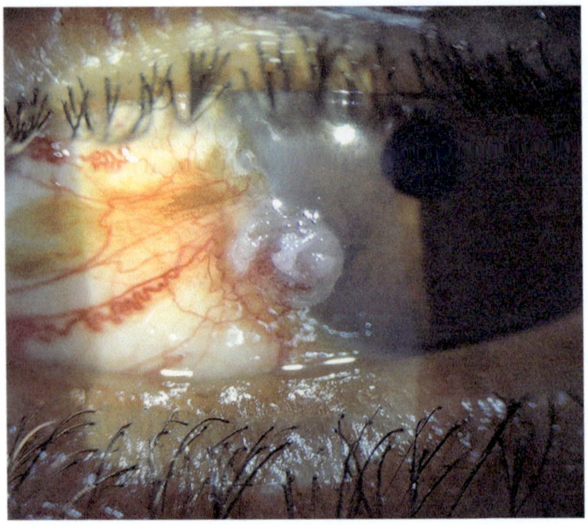

Gross slit lamp illumination image of the right eye of a patient depicting a 4 × 4 mm white silvery plaque-like mass abutting the temporal conjunctiva, limbus, and cornea at 8 o' clock, suggestive of ocular surface squamous neoplasia. A corkscrew vessel can also be seen

2.2.2 Nodular Mulberry-Shaped Lobulated OSSN

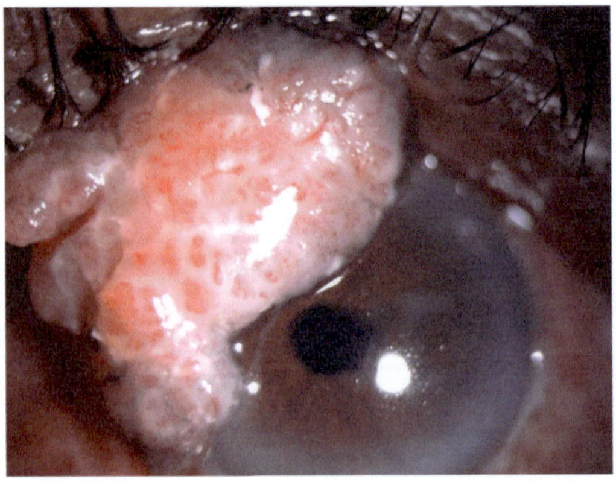

Gross slit lamp illumination image of the right eye of a patient depicting a mulberry-shaped elevated plaque abutting the temporal conjunctiva sclera, limbus, and cornea from 8 to 1 o' clock cornea, suggestive of ocular surface squamous neoplasia. The lesion is large, irregular, and exophytic, with a prominent, elevated, and fleshy appearance. It is located on the bulbar conjunctiva, extending over the limbus and encroaching onto the cornea. The surface of the lesion is highly vascularized, with visible dilated blood vessels, giving it a reddish, nodular appearance. The mass has a lobulated structure, and the surrounding conjunctiva appears inflamed, with some areas showing signs of congestion. The lesion's size and aggressive growth pattern suggest an advanced stage of OSSN, requiring prompt medical or surgical intervention

2.2.3 Corneal OSSN with Keratinization

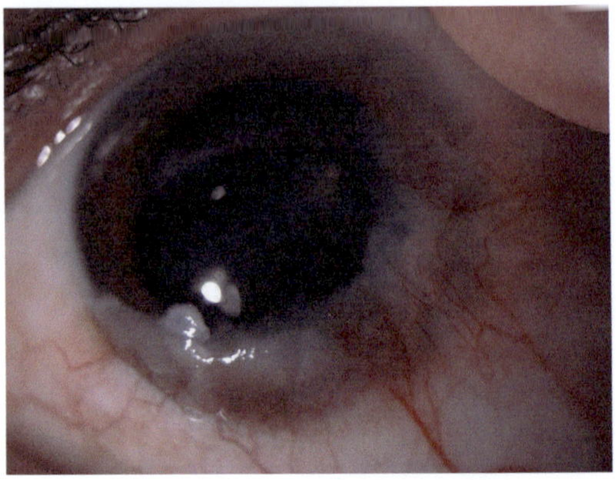

Diffuse illumination slit lamp image of the right eye of a patient depicting silvery plaque-shaped growth from 1 to 8 o' clock cornea abutting the limbus suggestive of ocular surface squamous neoplasia. Corkscrew vessels can also be made out. The OSSN is characterized by a thickened, elevated, and irregular lesion located primarily on the limbus and extending onto the cornea. The lesion appears opaque with a whitish hue, indicating keratinization or a dense accumulation of abnormal cells. The surrounding conjunctiva shows signs of vascularization, with visible blood vessels and mild congestion. The lesion has an irregular surface, suggesting an active proliferative process

2.2.4 OSSN with Conjunctival Naevus

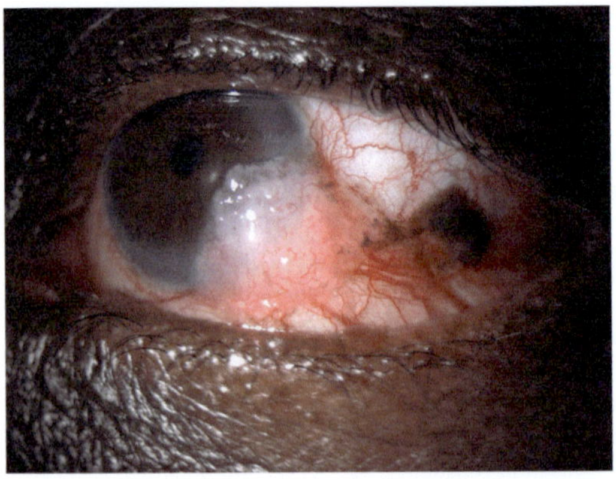

Gross slit lamp illumination image of the right eye of a patient depicting silvery elevated plaque abutting the nasal conjunctiva, limbus, and cornea from 3 to 5 o' clock cornea along with corkscrew vessels suggestive of ocular surface squamous neoplasia. A small pigmented conjunctival naevus can be made out adjacent to corkscrew vessels

2.3 Stevens-Johnson Syndrome

2.3.1 Lid Margin Keratinization

SJS is a severe mucocutaneous disorder often triggered by medications or infections, leading to widespread epithelial cell death. Ocular involvement includes severe conjunctivitis, corneal ulcers, and symblepharon formation, potentially leading to blindness. Management focuses on acute care with systemic immunosuppression and long-term ocular surface rehabilitation, including amniotic membrane transplantation and limbal stem cell transplantation [2].

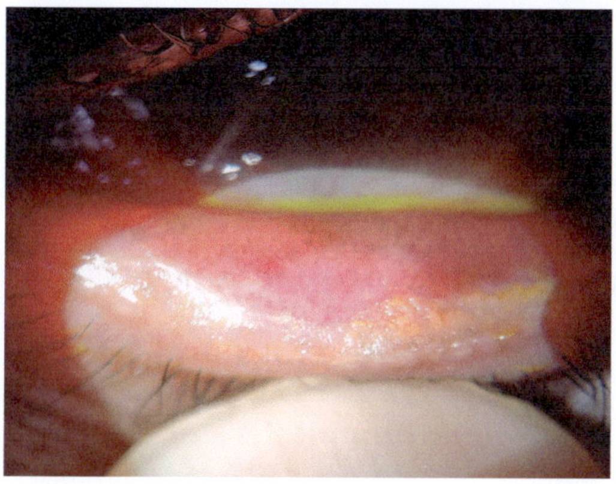

Gross slit lamp illumination image of a Stevens-Johnson syndrome patient's lower lid depicting keratinization along with inflamed lid margin

2.3.2 Severe Aqueous Deficiency Dry Eye

Severe aqueous deficiency dry eye (ADDE) is characterized by a significant reduction in tear production, leading to ocular surface inflammation and damage. This condition can result in deep corneal neovascularization as the eye attempts to compensate for the chronic dryness and inflammation by forming new blood vessels. Management includes aggressive lubrication, anti-inflammatory therapies, and possibly surgical interventions to address the neovascularization and restore ocular surface health [3].

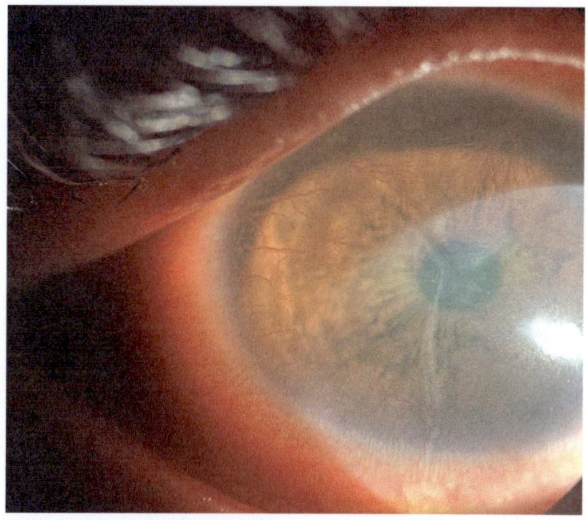

Digital illumination gross image of a patient's eye depicting meibomian gland plugging, diffuse conjunctival congestion, superficial corneal vascularization, and lusterless cornea suggestive of aqueous deficiency dry eye

2.4 Tenon's Patch Graft

2.4.1 Corneal Perforation Plugged with Tenon's Patch Graft

Tenon's patch graft is used in reconstructive surgery of the ocular surface, particularly in cases of corneal perforation. It provides a vascularized tissue that supports epithelial regeneration and prevents recurrence of scarring [4].

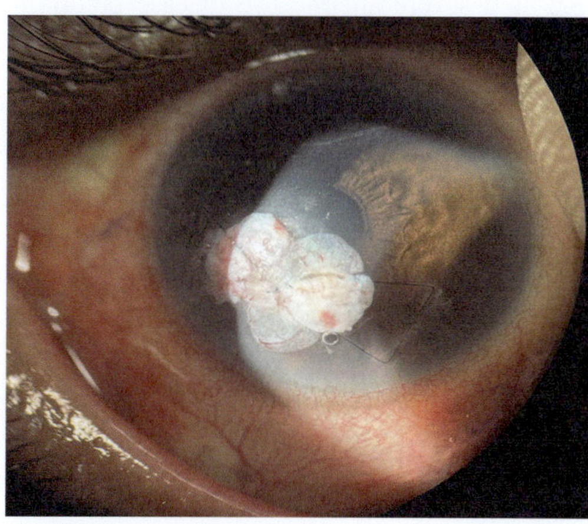

Gross slit lamp illumination image of a patient post Tenon's patch graft for small corneal perforation. The anterior chamber is well formed, and the sutures are well aligned holding the Tenon patch graft in place

2.4.2 Healed Cornea with Scar

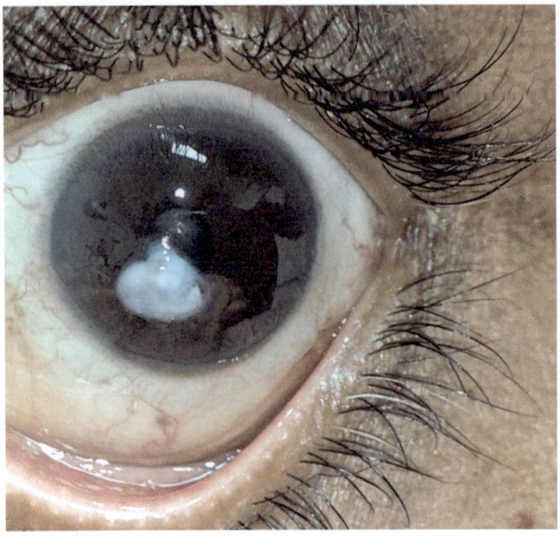

Gross illumination image of a patient post Tenon's patch graft for small corneal perforation in the case of herpes simplex keratitis. The anterior chamber is well formed post Tenon's patch graft

2.5 Vernal Keratoconjunctivitis

2.5.1 Severe Vernal Keratoconjunctivitis (VKC) with Limbal Stem Cell Deficiency

VKC is a severe allergic eye disease predominantly affecting young males. It presents with intense itching, photophobia, and thick mucus discharge. Treatment includes topical antihistamines, mast cell stabilizers, and corticosteroids. In severe cases, immunosuppressants and surgical interventions may be necessary [5]. Limbal stem cell deficiency (LSCD) occurs due to loss or dysfunction of limbal stem cells, essential for corneal epithelial regeneration. Causes include chemical injuries, Stevens-Johnson syndrome, and prolonged contact lens wear. Treatment involves limbal stem cell transplantation and adjunctive therapies to promote stem cell survival [6].

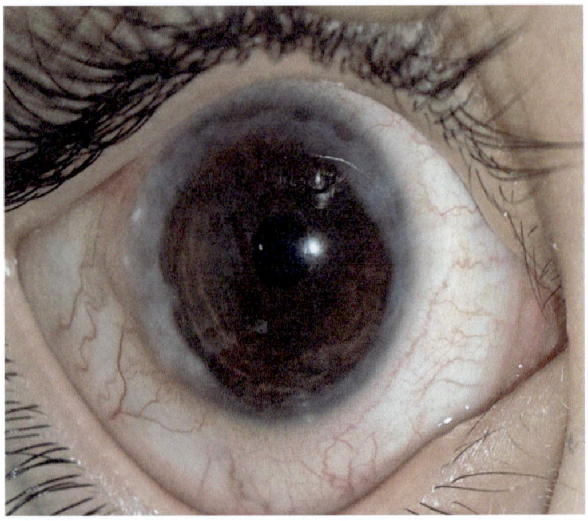

Diffuse illumination slit lamp image of a patient depicting total limbal stem cell deficiency with 360 degree Horner-Trantas spots suggestive of severe vernal keratoconjunctivitis

2.6 Neurotrophic Keratopathy

2.6.1 Neurotrophic Ulcer with Lagophthalmos

Neurotrophic keratopathy is characterized by decreased corneal sensitivity and poor epithelial healing due to impaired corneal innervation. It can be caused by herpes simplex virus, herpes zoster virus, diabetes, or trigeminal nerve damage. Treatment includes preservative-free artificial tears, therapeutic contact lenses, and recombinant human nerve growth factor (cenegermin) [7].

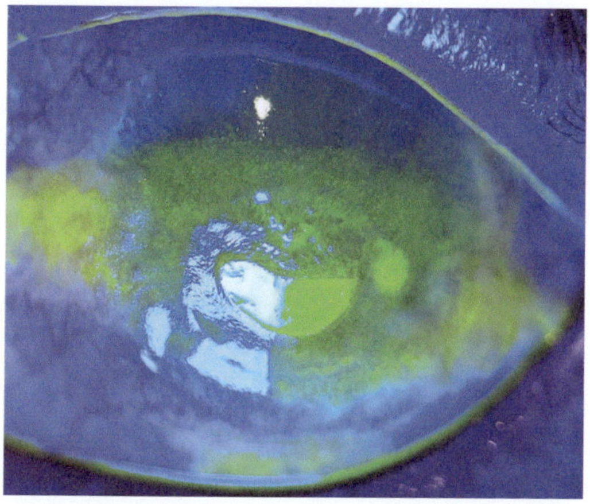

Diffuse illumination cobalt blue slit lamp image of a patient under fluorescent staining depicting diffuse punctate epithelial erosions, dry corneal surface, and central punched out corneal ulceration suggestive of neurotrophic keratitis in a patient with lagophthalmos

2.6.2 Neurotrophic Ulcer with Severe Corneal Thinning

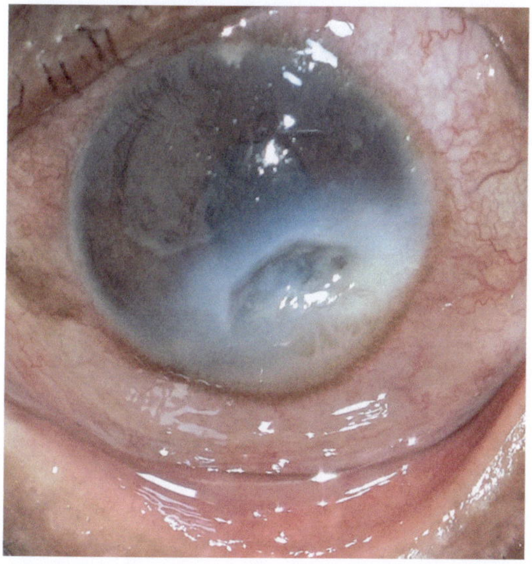

Diffuse illumination slit lamp image of a patient depicting diffuse conjunctival congestion, inferonasal half corneal scarring with excavated thinned out area of corneal ulceration suggestive of neurotrophic keratitis

2.7 Pterygium

2.7.1 Double Pterygium

Pterygium is a fibrovascular growth of the conjunctiva onto the cornea, often associated with UV exposure. It can cause irritation, dryness, and visual impairment. Treatment involves surgical excision, often combined with conjunctival autografting or amniotic membrane transplantation to reduce recurrence [8].

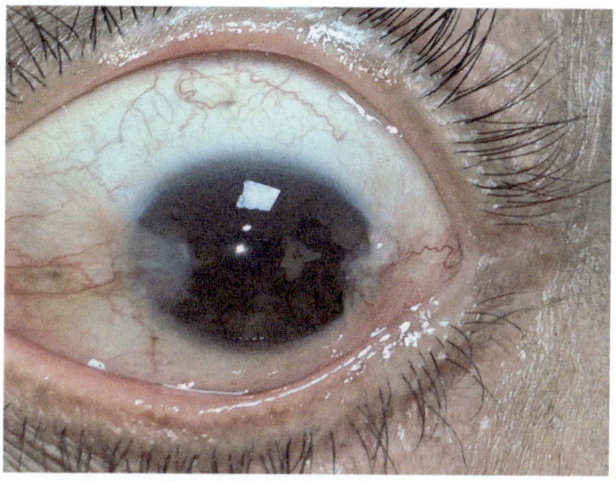

Diffuse illumination slit lamp image of a patient depicting nasal and temporal fleshy pterygium with wettability of the ocular surface

2.8 Meibomitis

2.8.1 Severe Meibomitis

Meibomitis, or meibomian gland dysfunction (MGD), involves inflammation of the meibomian glands, leading to tear film instability and evaporative dry eye. Management includes warm compresses, lid hygiene, and systemic or topical antibiotics [9].

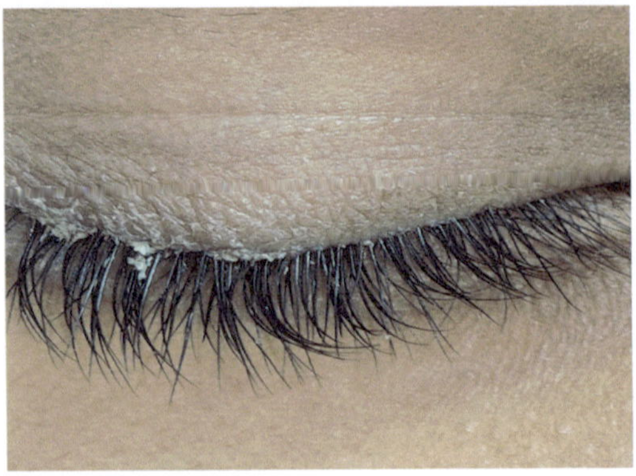

Diffuse illumination gross image of a patient depicting meibomitis and blepharitis with crusting

2.8.2 Pyogenic Granuloma

Pyogenic granuloma is a benign vascular lesion that can occur on the conjunctiva following trauma or surgery. Treatment involves topical or intralesional corticosteroids and, in persistent cases, surgical excision [10].

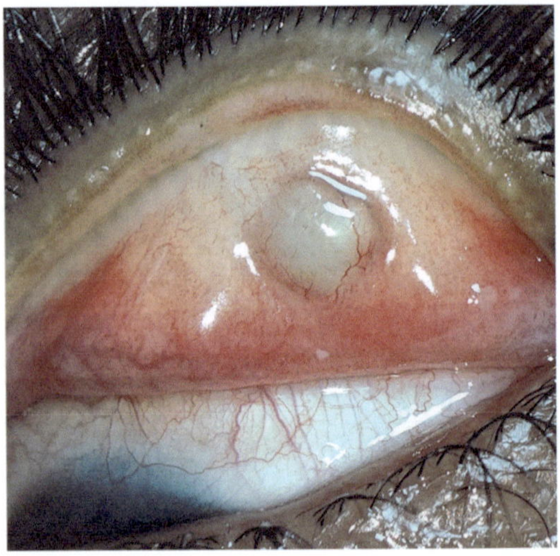

Diffuse illumination slit lamp image of a patient depicting granuloma in the upper tarsal conjunctiva

2.9 Corneal Scarring

2.9.1 Corneal Scar with Band-Shaped Keratopathy

Corneal scarring can result from trauma, infection, or surgery, leading to visual impairment. Treatment options include phototherapeutic keratectomy (PTK) and, in severe cases, corneal transplantation [11]. Band-shaped keratopathy is characterized by the deposition of calcium in the superficial cornea, often associated with chronic inflammation or systemic metabolic disorders. Treatment includes chelation therapy with EDTA and, in advanced cases, superficial keratectomy [11].

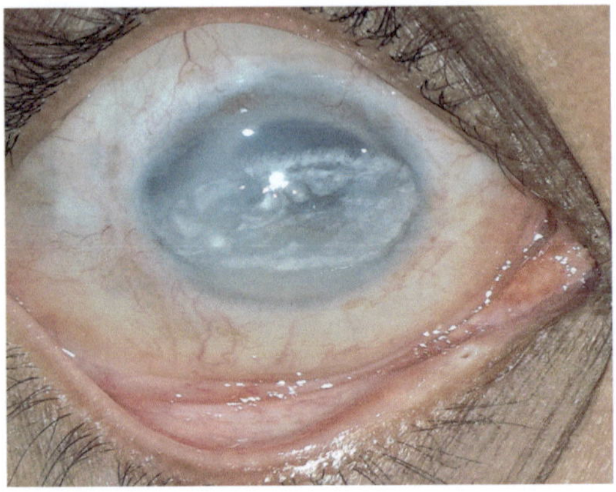

Diffuse illumination slit lamp image of a patient depicting horizontal central corneal scar with band-shaped keratopathy in an absolute eye post-trauma

2.10 Superior Limbic Keratoconjunctivitis (SLK)

2.10.1 Superior Limbic Keratoconjunctivitis with Conjunctival Chemosis

SLK is a chronic inflammatory condition primarily affecting the superior conjunctiva and cornea. It often presents with redness, foreign body sensation, and irritation. SLK is frequently associated with thyroid dysfunction, particularly hyperthyroidism. The management includes lubricants, anti-inflammatory medications, and in refractory cases, surgical resection of the affected conjunctiva [12].

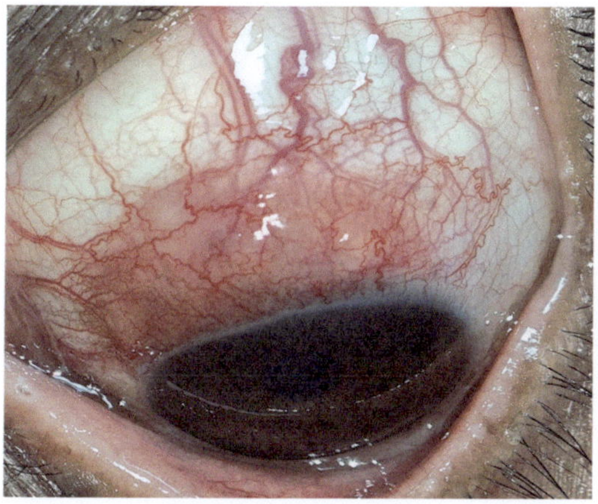

Diffuse illumination slit lamp image of a patient with superior limbic keratoconjunctivitis. In downgaze, there is superior conjunctival chemosis along with congestion in the superior quadrant

2.10.2 Uveal Tissue Prolapse

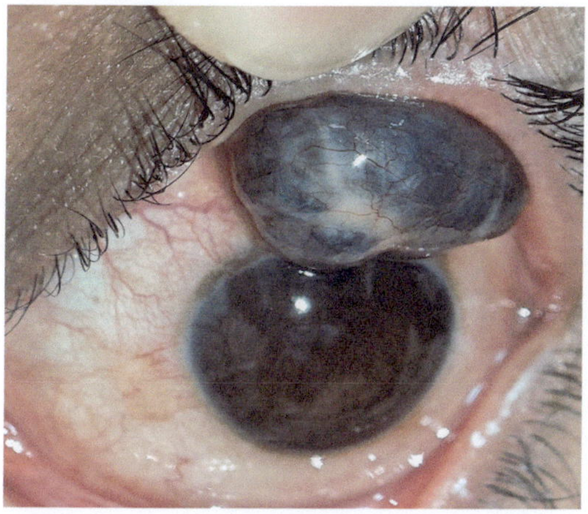

Diffuse illumination slit lamp image of the patient depicting uveal tissue prolapse well epithelialized with conjunctiva from the superior quadrant suggestive of old scleromalacia perforans

2.11 Chemical Injury

2.11.1 Dua's Classification Grade 3

Chemical injuries to the eye can cause severe damage to the cornea and conjunctiva, leading to vision loss. Immediate irrigation is crucial, followed by medical and surgical interventions to manage inflammation and promote healing [13].

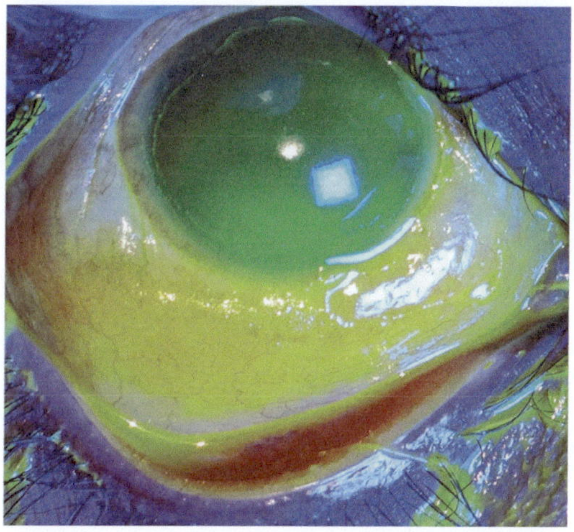

Diffuse illumination slit lamp image of a patient with chemical injury depicting conjunctival staining, inferior forniceal subconjunctival hemorrhage, and total corneal epithelial defect with corneal staining with limbal ischemia

2.11.2 Dua's Classification Grade 5

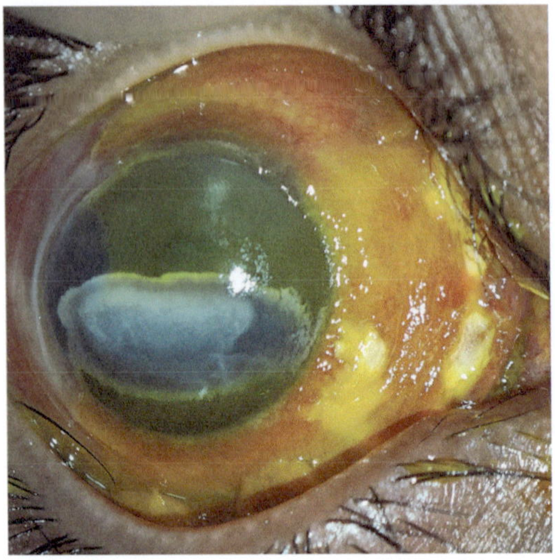

Diffuse illumination slit lamp image of a patient depicting conjunctival blanching with ulceration and large corneal epithelial defect with oval-shaped deposit of lime in the central and inferior half of the cornea sparing the limbus

2.11.3 Corneal Scar, Symblepharon, and Vascularization

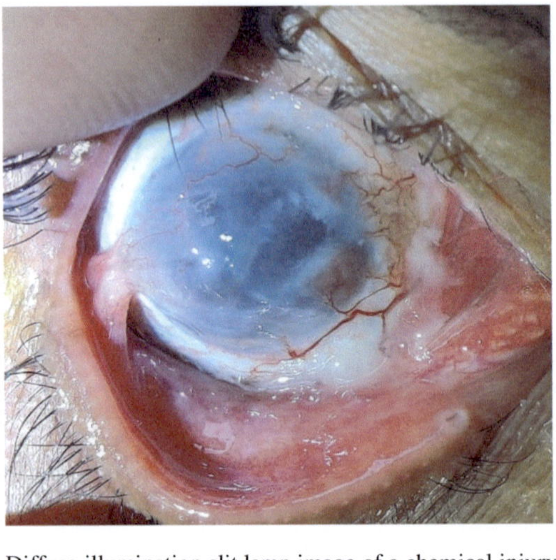

Diffuse illumination slit lamp image of a chemical injury patient depicting inflamed conjunctiva, temporal symblepharon, total corneal scarring with thinning, and superficial and deep corneal vascularization

2.11.4 Neurotrophic Ulcer

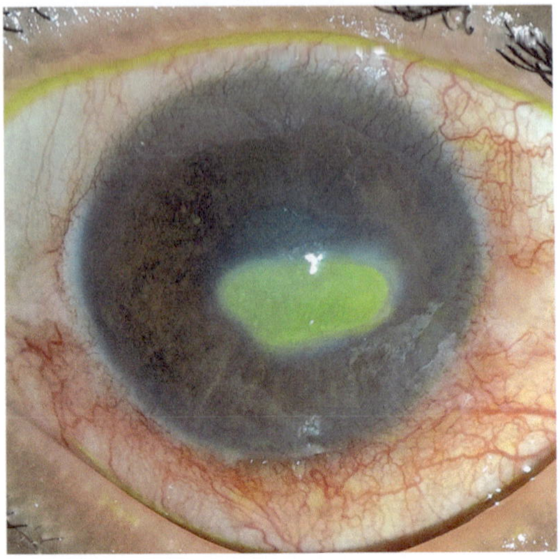

Diffuse illumination slit lamp image of a patient depicting circumciliary congestion along with central punched out corneal ulcer under fluorescein staining suggestive of neurotrophic keratitis

2.11.5 Dellen

Dellen are localized corneal thinning adjacent to raised lesions or scars, leading to tear film instability and epithelial breakdown. Treatment involves addressing the underlying cause, using lubricants and therapeutic contact lenses [14].

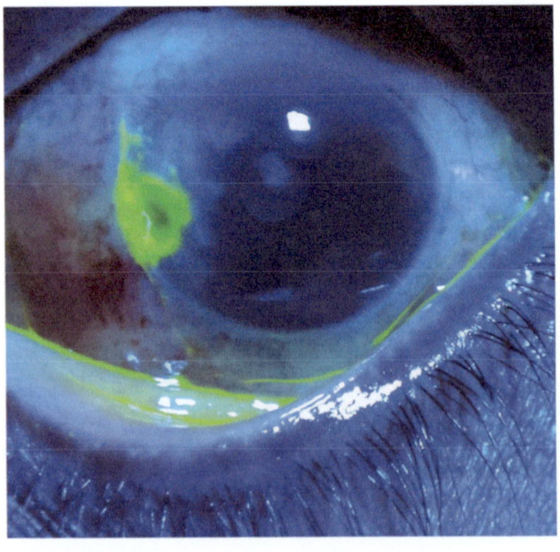

Diffuse illumination cobalt blue filter slit lamp image of a patient depicting dellen at 9 o' clock cornea under fluorescein staining post-pterygium surgery

2.12 Pterygium

2.12.1 Inflamed Pterygium

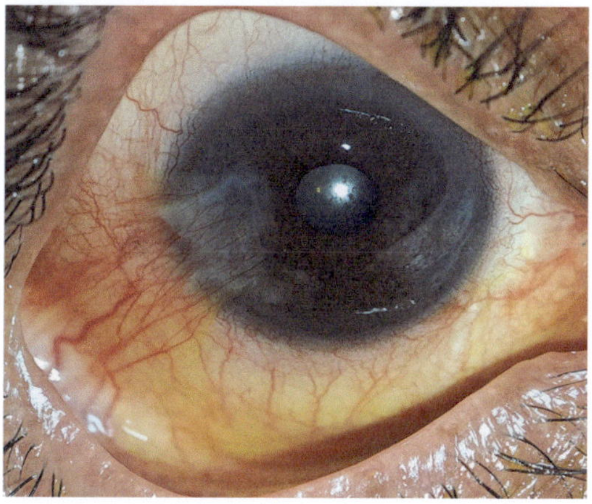

Diffuse illumination slit lamp image of a patient depicting inflamed fleshy temporal pterygium

2.12.2 Spillover Glue Over the Pterygium Graft

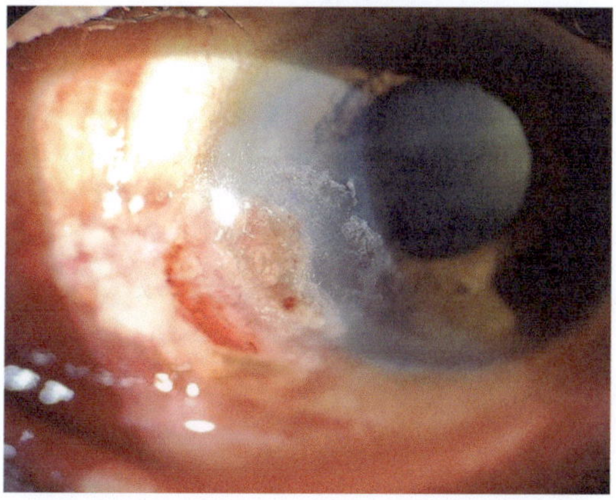

Diffuse illumination slit lamp image of a patient depicting spillover glue over the temporal cornea from the conjunctival autograft

2.12.3 Vascularized Corneal Opacity

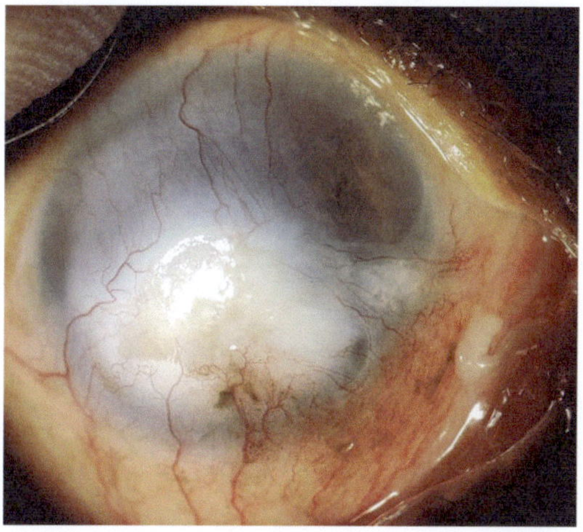

Diffuse illumination slit lamp image of a patient depicting nasal conjunctival congestion, near-total limbal stem cell deficiency, fibrovascular pannus, and leukomatous corneal scar in a patient post-herpes viral keratitis

2.12.4 Anterior Staphyloma

Anterior staphyloma is the protrusion of uveal tissue through a weakened cornea, often following severe inflammation or trauma. Management involves surgical reconstruction, including corneal grafting or scleral reinforcement [15].

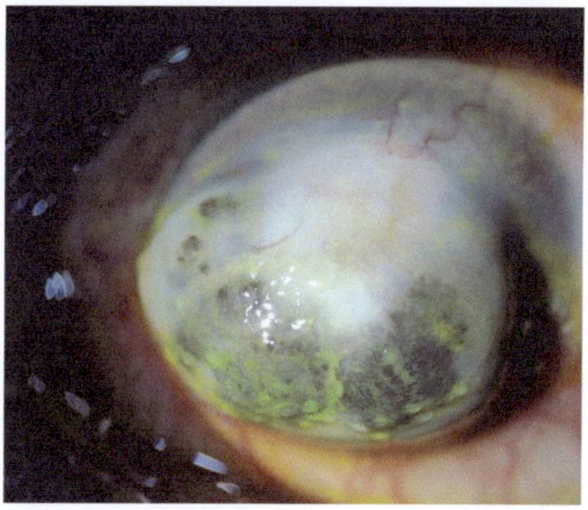

Diffuse illumination slit lamp image of a post-trauma patient depicting anterior staphyloma with corneal scar and uveal tissue

2.13 Post-Full Thickness Keratoplasty

2.13.1 Poor Epithelialization

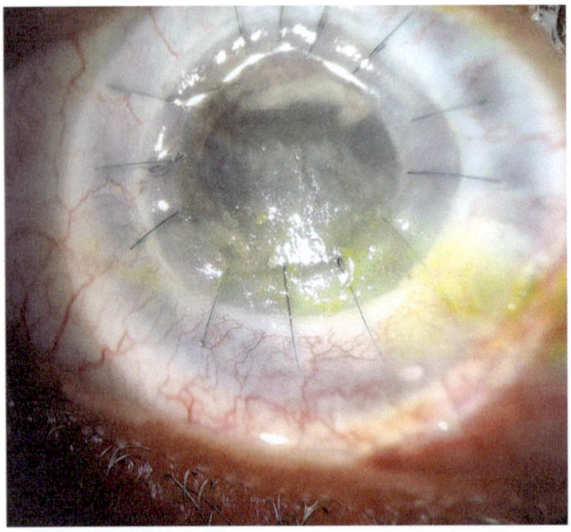

Diffuse illumination slit lamp image of a patient depicting host corneal vascularization, 8 mm corneal graft with poor epithelialization, well-opposed graft host junction, intact suture with adequate tightness, and dilated 8 mm pupil with aphakia

2.13.2 Auto-Evisceration

Auto evisceration refers to the spontaneous extrusion of intraocular contents, usually following severe infection or trauma. It requires immediate surgical intervention to repair and reconstruct the ocular surface [16].

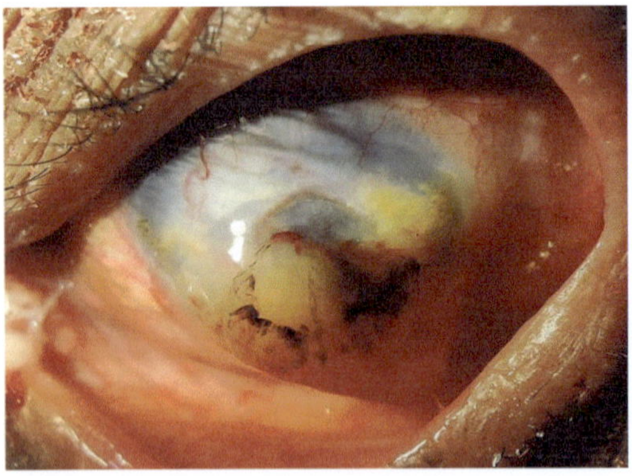

Diffuse illumination slit lamp image of a corneal ulcer patient depicting auto-evisceration in a case of long-standing cornel perforation

2.13.3 Limbal Stem Cell Deficiency with Pannus

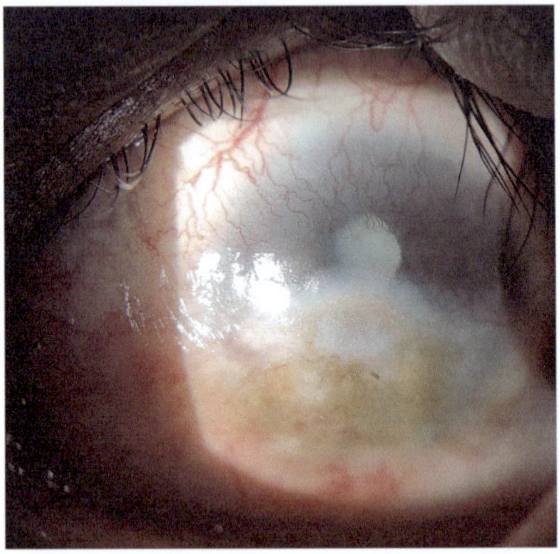

Diffuse slit lamp image of a patient depicting total limbal stem cell deficiency, superior 180 degree corneal neovascularization, and pannus in inferior half of the cornea

2.13.4 Corneal Ulcer

Corneal ulcers are open sores on the cornea, typically resulting from infection. Prompt diagnosis and treatment with antibiotics, antifungals, or antivirals are essential to prevent vision loss [17].

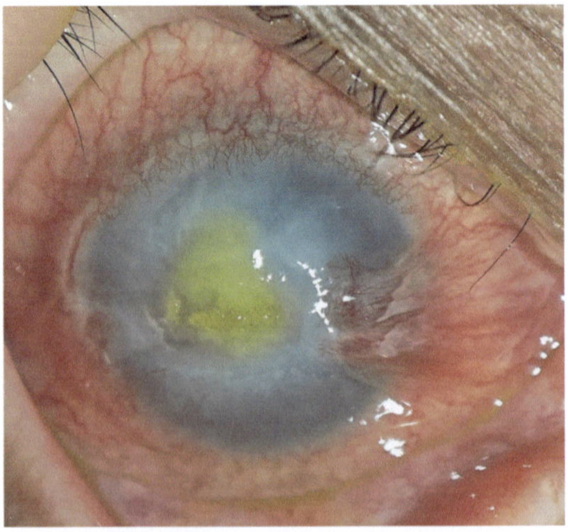

Diffuse slit lamp image of a patient depicting diffuse conjunctival congestion and inflamed nasal pterygium with healing of the central 4 × 4 mm corneal ulcer

2.13.5 Conjunctival Granuloma over Cornea

Conjunctival granulomas are inflammatory lesions that can occur following infection, trauma, or surgery. Treatment involves corticosteroids and, if necessary, surgical excision [18].

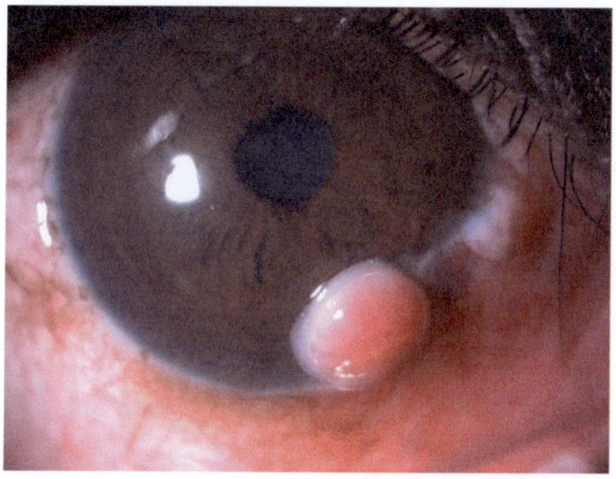

Diffuse illumination slit lamp image of a patient depicting conjunctival granuloma over the cornea at 5 o' clock position abutting the limbus

References

1. Galor A, Karp CL, Oellers P, Kao AA, Abdelaziz A, Feuer W, et al. Predictors of ocular surface squamous neoplasia recurrence after excisional surgery. Ophthalmology. 2012;119(2):197–203.
2. Mimura T, Yamagami S, Usui T, Funatsu H, Mimura Y, Noma H, et al. Conjunctivochalasis: association with higher ages and nasal location. Ophthalmology. 2016;123(2):403–11.
3. Messmer EM. The pathophysiology, diagnosis, and treatment of dry eye disease. Dtsch Arztebl Int. 2015;112(5):71–82.
4. Ahmad S. Concise review: limbal stem cell deficiency, dysfunction, and distress. Stem Cells Transl Med. 2012;1(2):110–5.
5. Bonini S, Coassin M, Aronni S, Lambiase A. Vernal keratoconjunctivitis. Eye (Lond). 2004;18(4):345–51.
6. Grostern RJ, Ta CN. External ocular infections. Curr Opin Ophthalmol. 2010;21(4):331–5.
7. Krachmer JH, Mannis MJ, Holland EJ. Cornea. Elsevier Health Sciences; 2013. Chapter 174: 2083-2084
8. Chui J, Coroneo MT, Tat LT, Crouch R, Wakefield D, Di Girolamo N. Ophthalmic pterygium: a stem cell disorder with premalignant features. Am J Pathol. 2011;178(2):817–27.
9. Geerling G, Tauber J, Baudouin C, Goto E, Matsumoto Y, O'Brien T, et al. The international workshop on Meibomian gland dysfunction: report of the subcommittee on management and treatment of Meibomian gland dysfunction. Invest Ophthalmol Vis Sci. 2011;52(4):2050–64.
10. Eltahir AM, Mohammed MA, Yousif MA. Pyogenic granuloma of the conjunctiva: a case report. J Med Case Rep. 2014;8:112.
11. Rajasekaran S, D'Aversa G, Starr CE. Management of band keratopathy and calcific scleral plaque. Curr Opin Ophthalmol. 2015;26(4):281–7.
12. Kinoshita S, Yokoi N, Komuro A. Recent advances in superior limbic keratoconjunctivitis. Eye Contact Lens. 2015;41(5):229–31.
13. Sharma N, Kaur M, Agarwal T, Sangwan VS, Vajpayee RB. Treatment of acute ocular chemical burns. Surv Ophthalmol. 2018;63(2):214–35.
14. Liang L, Sheha H, Tseng SC. Surgical management of chronic Stevens-Johnson syndrome. Ocul Surf. 2016;14(1):11–9.
15. Lewis EJ, Finger PT. Anterior staphyloma: a clinical perspective. Int Ophthalmol Clin. 2018;58(2):113–22.
16. Qureshi MH, Laghari K, Lakhair MA. Management of auto-evisceration in neglected severe chemical burn of eye. J Ayub Med Coll Abbottabad. 2017;29(3):509–11.
17. Eltis M. Infectious keratitis and contact lens wear: a review. Cont Lens Anterior Eye. 2018;41(1):47–51.
18. López-Gálvez MI, Sáez-Escudero E, López-Sánchez E, Pastor-Vivas AI, Cordero-Coma M, Méndez-Vila C. Giant conjunctival granuloma: a case report. BMC Ophthalmol. 2017;17(1):169.

Ocular Surface Diseases

3

Shweta Agarwal, Bhaskar Srinivasan, and Geetha Iyer

3.1 Introduction

Ocular surface diseases encompass a broad array of conditions affecting the conjunctiva and cornea, often leading to significant visual impairment and discomfort. These diseases can arise from various etiologies, including inflammatory, infectious, traumatic, and autoimmune origins. Understanding these conditions is crucial for implementing effective treatment strategies to preserve vision and improve patient outcomes. This chapter explores several key ocular surface diseases and their management, including pterygium, autologous conjunctival transplantation, limbal stem cell transplantation, mucous membrane grafts, persistent corneal epithelial defects, chemical injury, corneal thinning and perforation, Boston keratoprosthesis, tarsorrhaphy, corneal tattooing, Stevens-Johnson syndrome, vernal keratoconjunctivitis, shield ulcer, ocular cicatricial pemphigoid, and neurotrophic ulcer.

3.2 Limbal Stem Cell Deficiency (LSCD)

3.2.1 Total Limbal Stem Cell Deficiency (LSCD) with Limbal Stem Cell Transplantation

Limbal stem cell deficiency (LSCD) can lead to persistent epithelial defects, conjunctivalization of the cornea, and vision loss. Limbal stem cell transplantation, using autologous or allogeneic sources, aims to restore the limbal stem cell population, essential for corneal epithelial regeneration. This technique is often combined with amniotic membrane transplantation to enhance outcomes [1, 2].

S. Agarwal (✉) · B. Srinivasan · G. Iyer
CJ Shah Cornea Services, Medical Research Foundation, Sankara Nethralaya, Chennai, Tamil Nadu, India

B. Gurnani, K. Kaur (eds.), *Atlas of Cornea*, https://doi.org/10.1007/978-981-96-0013-7_3

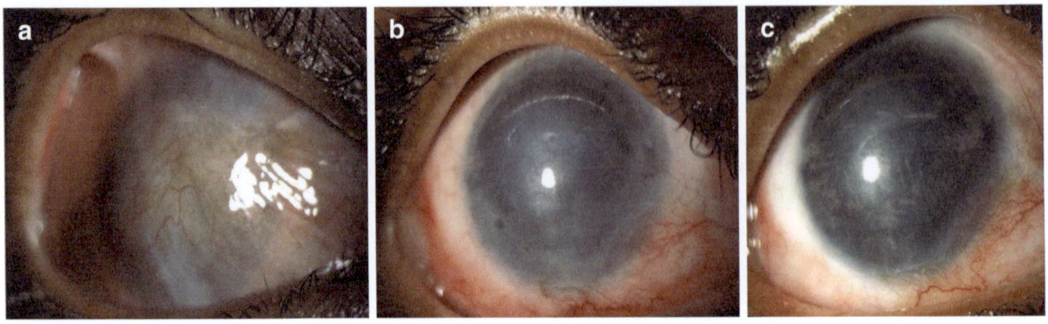

(**a**) Diffuse illumination slit lamp image of the right eye depicting total limbal stem cell deficiency 7 months following chemical injury with grade 1–2 symblepharon. (**b**) 1 month following auto-simple limbal epithelial transplant (SLET) with symblepharon release+ amniotic membrane transplant (AMT), epithelialized surface with corneal phenotype and well-formed fornices. (**c**) Stable surface with a gradual reduction in the density of corneal scar, 3 years following auto-SLET

3.2.2 Surface Keratinization

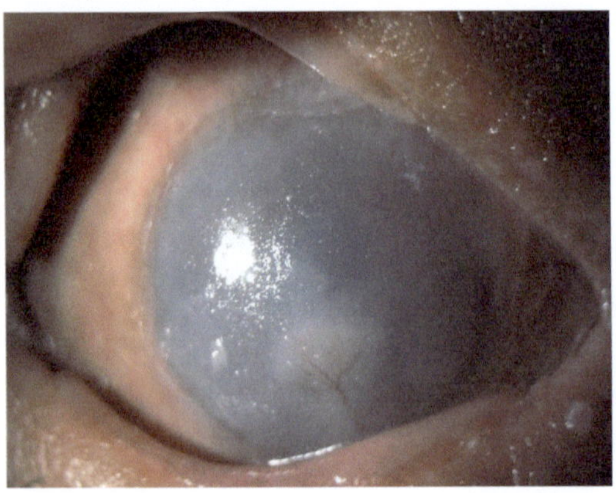

Diffuse illumination slit lamp image of a patient with limbal stem cell deficiency with early surface keratinization

3.2.3 Dry Keratinized Surface

Dry keratinized surface with limbal stem cell deficiency (LSCD) occurs when the loss of limbal stem cells leads to the failure of corneal epithelium maintenance, resulting in conjunctivalization, neovascularization, and keratinization of the corneal surface. This condition severely impairs vision and requires strategies such as limbal stem cell transplantation and ocular surface reconstruction to restore a healthy ocular surface [3].

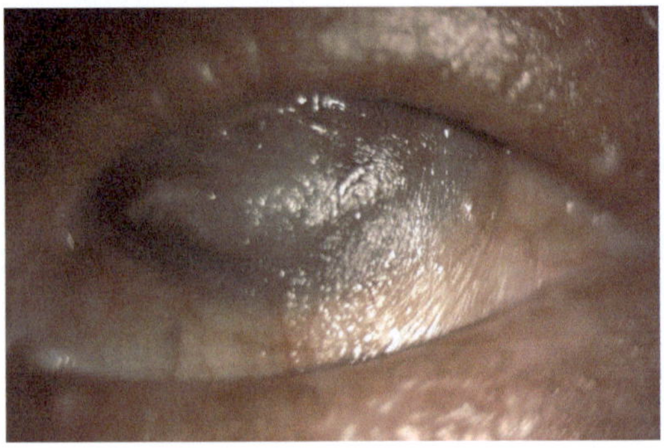

Dry keratinized surface with no view of the anterior chamber

3.2.4 Partial and Total LSCD

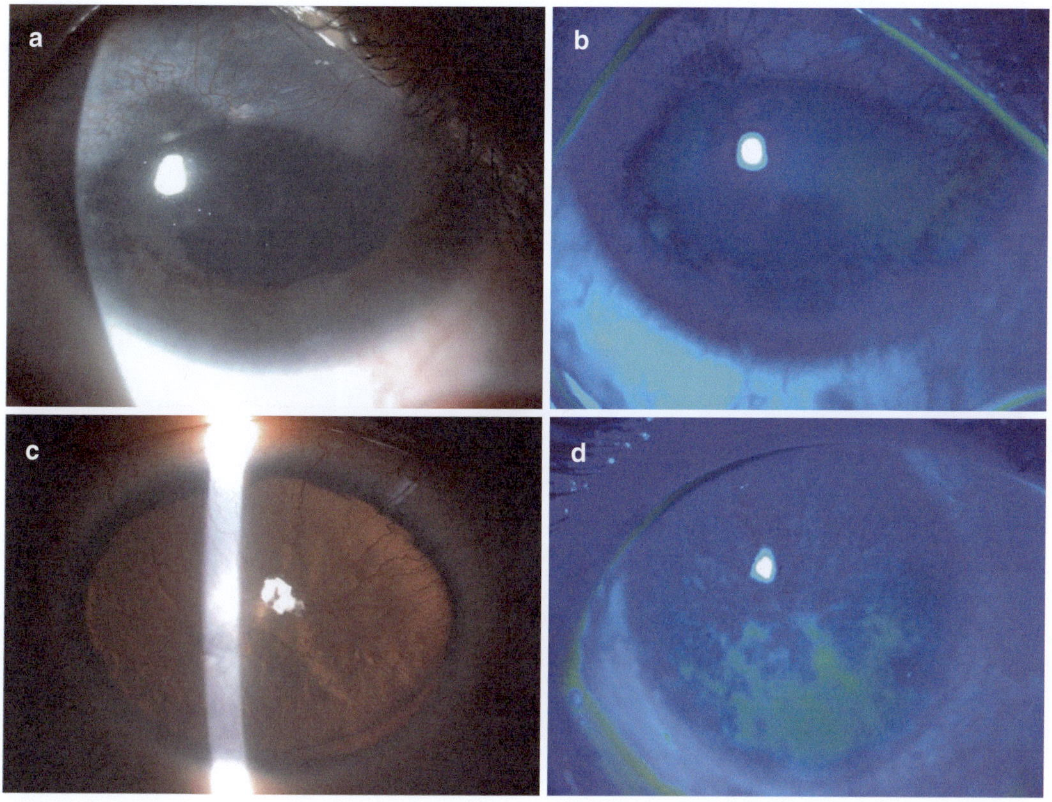

Diffuse illumination slit lamp image of a patient depicting. (**a**, **b**) partial LSCD: peripheral 360-degree conjunctivalization of the cornea sparing the central area. Fluorescein stain showing a delayed conjunctival stippled staining corresponding to the peripheral area of conjunctivalization. (**c**, **d**) Total LSCD: 360-degree corneal vascularization in aniridia. Fluorescein stain showing a delayed conjunctival stippled staining of the entire corneal surface

3.2.5 Limbal Stem Cell Transplant

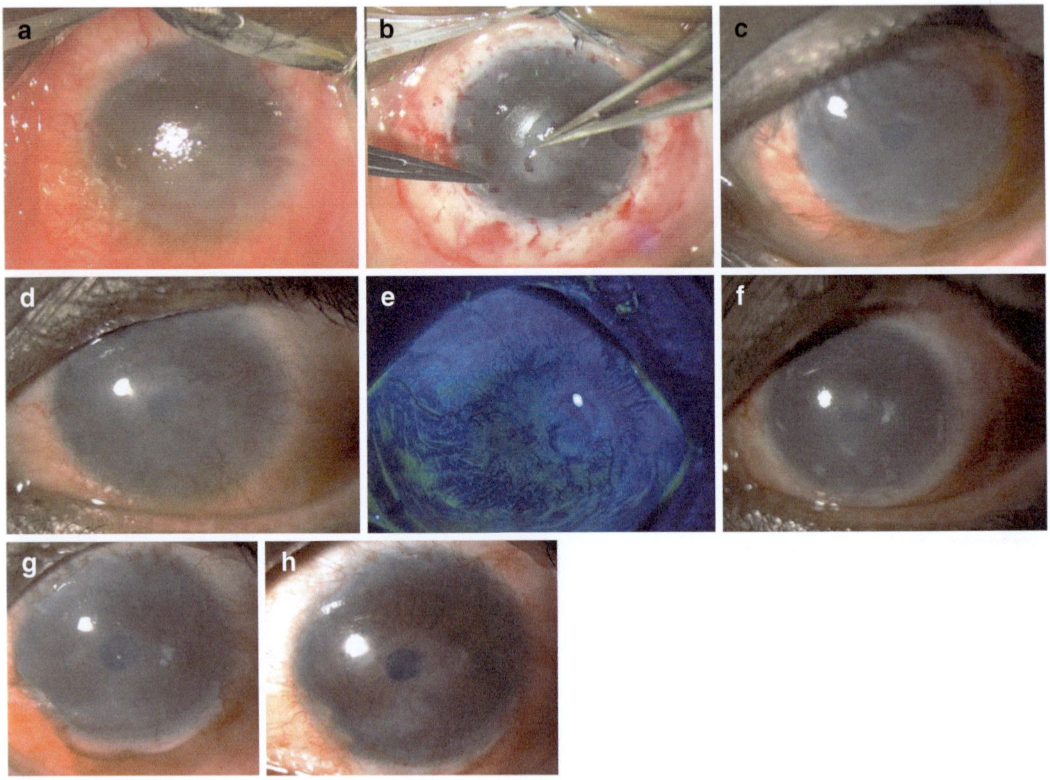

Limbal Stem Cell Transplant
Diffuse illumination slit lamp images of the patient depicting: (**a**) Total LSCD 8 months following chemical injury. (**b**) Pannus removal followed by anchoring of auto-SLET bits with fibrin glue over the amniotic membrane. (**c**) Epithelialized surface with a clear corneal phenotype, 1 month following auto-SLET. (**d**) Recurrence of limbal deficiency in the form of conjunctivalization noted 6 months following auto-SLET. (**e**) Fluorescein staining showing conjunctival phenotype indicating stem cell transplant failure. (**f**) Epithelialized surface, 2 weeks following re-auto-SLET. (**g**) 6 months following re-auto-SLET, a stable surface with corneal phenotype. (**h**) 3 years following re-auto-SLET, a stable surface with corneal phenotype with no evidence of recurrence

3.2.6 Allo-Simple Limbal Epithelial Transplant

Allo-simple limbal epithelial transplant (allo-SLET) involves transplanting limbal epithelial cells from a donor to the recipient's eye to restore the limbal stem cell population. This procedure is used to treat limbal stem cell deficiency, aiming to regenerate a healthy corneal epithelium and improve vision [4].

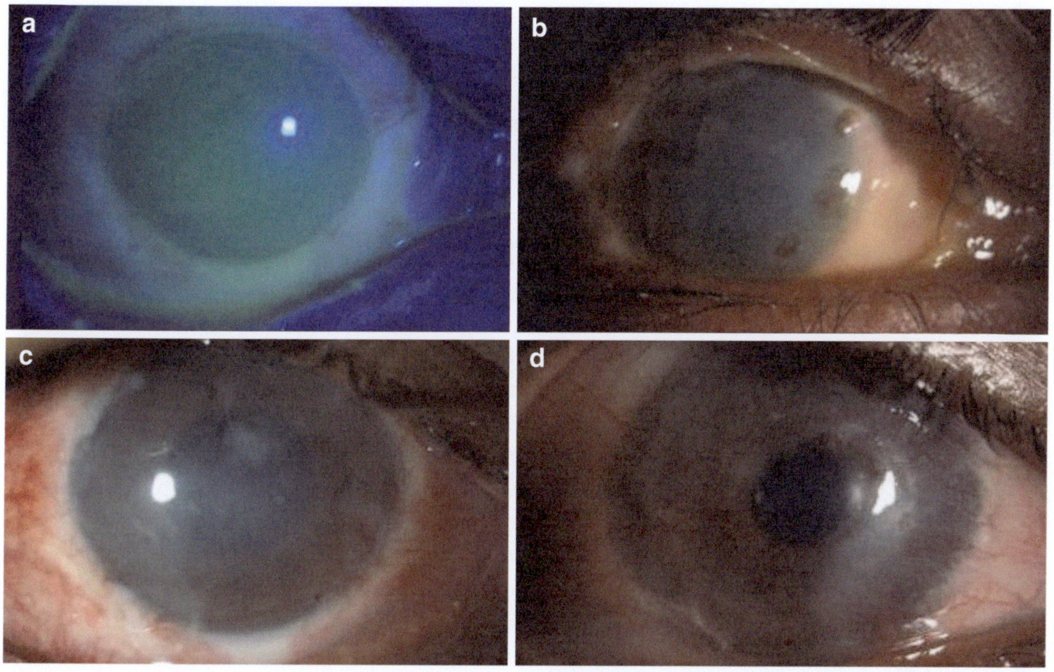

Diffuse illumination slit lamp image of the patient depicting: (**a**) Total epithelial defect in a 22-year-old person; 3 days following Dua's grade 6 chemical injury. (**b**) Slit lamp picture showing allo-SLET bits placed over an amniotic membrane to facilitate epithelialization in the acute stage. (**c**) Completely epithelialized surface noted 5 weeks following allo-SLET with a few retained bits. (**d**) Partial LSCD with central clear corneal phenotype, 7 months following allo-SLET, maintaining a vision of 20/80 without any further surgical intervention

3.2.7 Optical Keratoplasty with Keratolimbal Graft

Optical keratoplasty combined with a keratolimbal graft is a surgical technique used to treat severe limbal stem cell deficiency. This procedure involves transplanting both the corneal and limbal tissues to restore the ocular surface and improve visual acuity by addressing both the corneal opacity and the deficiency of limbal stem cells [5].

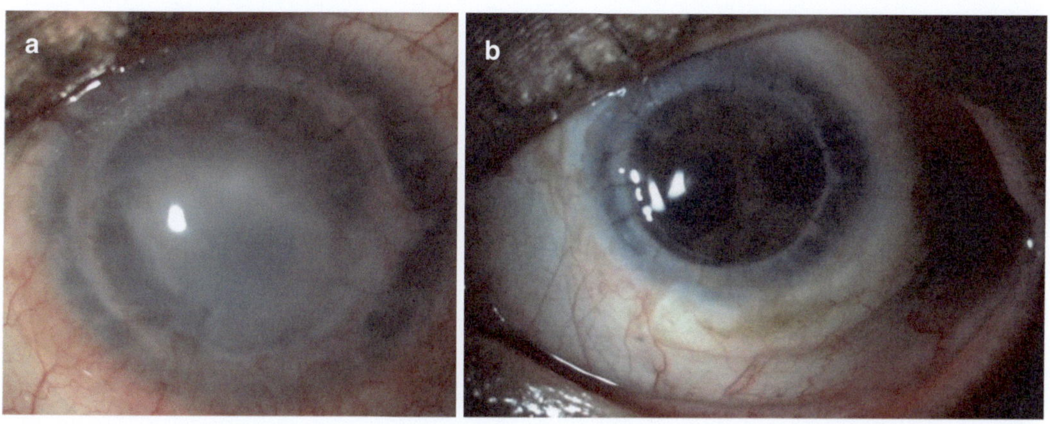

Diffuse illumination slit lamp image of a patient depicting: (**a**) One-eyed patient with failed vascularized graft following multiple keratoplasty in a moist eye. (**b**) 1 year following optical keratoplasty with keratolimbal allograft on oral immunosuppressive therapy maintaining clear graft with a stable surface

3.2.8 Boston Type 1 Keratoprosthesis

The Boston keratoprosthesis (KPro) is an artificial cornea used in patients with severe corneal opacification unresponsive to traditional keratoplasty. It provides a clear optical pathway, significantly improving vision in patients with end-stage corneal diseases [12].

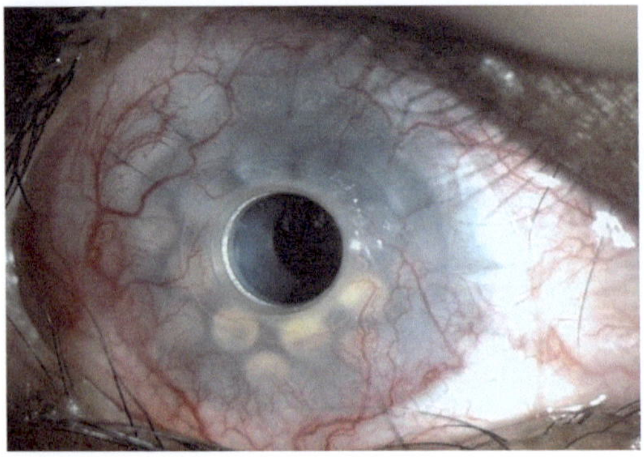

Diffuse illumination slit lamp image of a patient depicting well-fitted Type 1 Boston keratoprosthesis in a patient with 5-year post-chemical injury

3.3 Pterygium

3.3.1 Nasal, Temporal, and Double Pterygium

Pterygium is a common ocular surface condition characterized by a fibrovascular growth extending from the conjunctiva onto the cornea, often attributed to chronic UV exposure. It can cause visual impairment and discomfort, necessitating surgical excision. Adjunctive treatments, such as conjunctival autografting or amniotic membrane transplantation, help reduce recurrence rates [6].

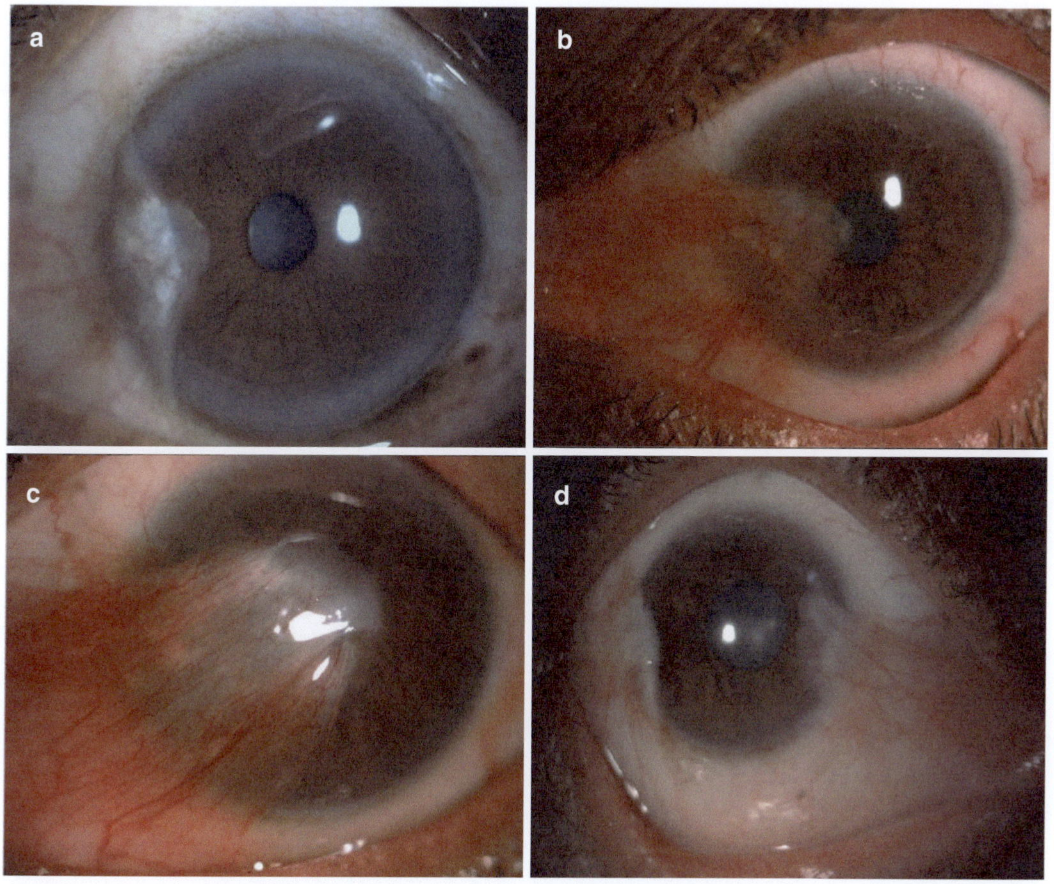

Diffuse illumination slit lamp image of different patients depicting: (**a**) Atrophic pterygium—can be observed; (**b**) progressive pterygium just reaching the visual axis—requires excision+ conjunctival autograft; (**c**) progressive pterygium obscuring the visual axis—requires excision+amniotic membrane transplant + conjunctival autograft; (**d**) dual pterygium—requires excision+ amniotic membrane transplant + conjunctival autograft

3.3.2 Recurrence and Post-Excision

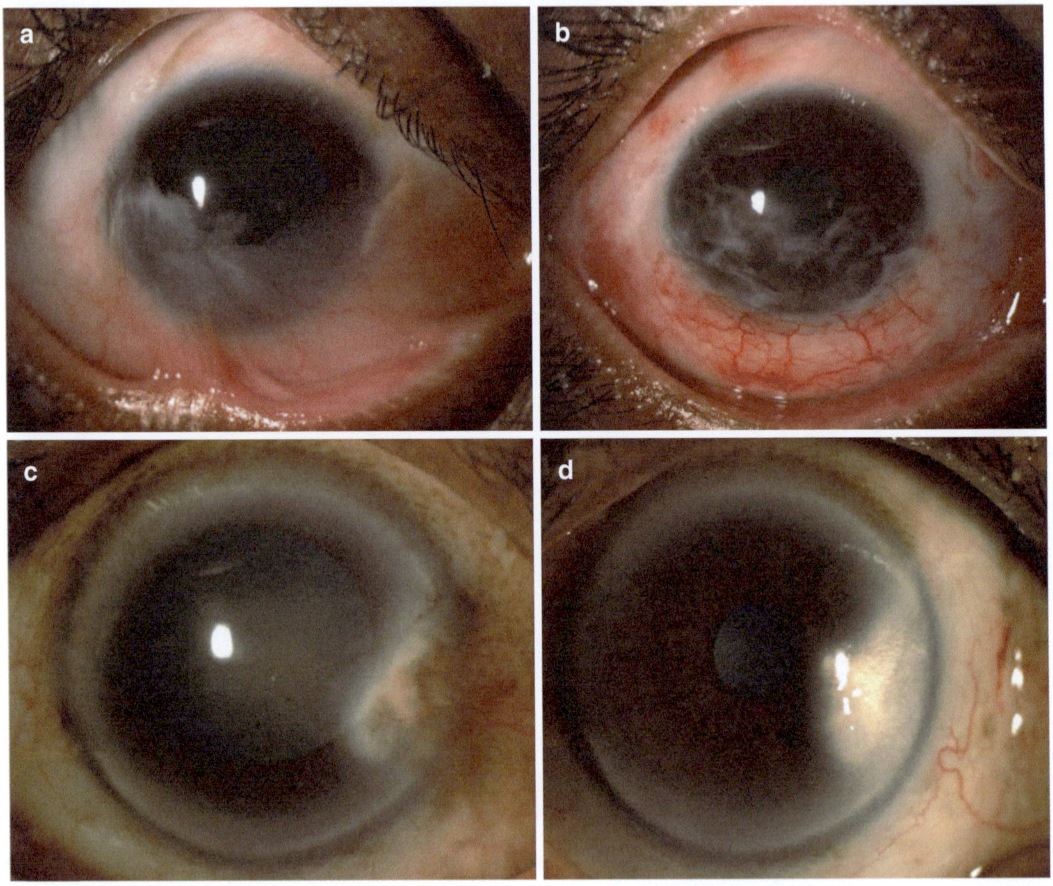

Diffuse illumination slit lamp image of a patient depicting: (**a**) Recurrent pterygium encroaching the visual axis partially. (**b**) 1 month following pterygium excision with conjunctival autograft and amniotic membrane transplant. (**c**) Long-standing pterygium with underlying scarring. (**d**) 6 months following pterygium excision along with conjunctival autograft

3.3.3 Persistent Epithelial Defect

Persistent corneal epithelial defects (PCEDs) result from various conditions, including neurotrophic keratopathy and dry eye disease. These nonhealing defects require treatments such as lubricants, therapeutic contact lenses, and surgical interventions like amniotic membrane transplantation to promote healing and restore corneal integrity [7, 8].

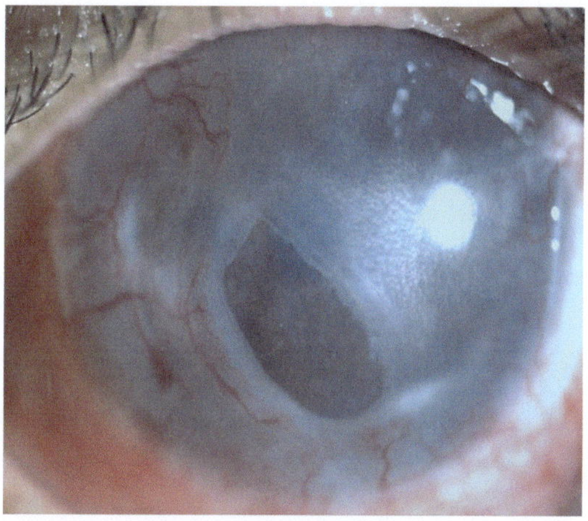

Diffuse illumination slit lamp image of a patient depicting persistent epithelial defect noted 3 months following Dua's grade 5 chemical injury despite multiple amniotic membrane transplants

3.4 Chemical Injury

3.4.1 Mild Chemical Injury

Chemical injuries to the eye can cause severe damage to the cornea and conjunctiva, leading to vision loss. Immediate irrigation is critical, followed by medical and surgical treatments to manage inflammation and promote healing. Interventions may include amniotic membrane transplantation and limbal stem cell transplantation [9].

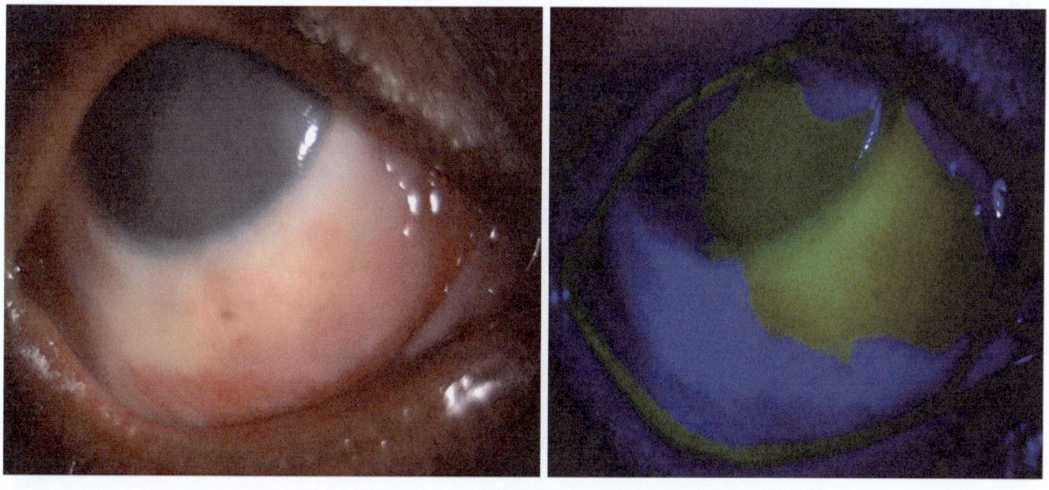

Diffuse illumination slit lamp image of a patient depicting

- Mild chemical injury involving less than 50% of cornea and 4 clock hours of limbus with 25% of conjunctival defect; no evidence of ischemia exposure
- EPIX classification of acute chemical injury: unilateral grade 2: E1-P0/I0/X0 [L2,C1, K1, T0]
- E—epithelial defect (L—limbal, C—conjunctival, K—Corneal, T—tarsal)
- P—intraocular pressure
- I—ischemia
- X—exposure

3.4.2 Moderate–Severe Grade of Chemical Injury

Moderate-to-severe grades of chemical injury to the eye can result in extensive damage to the cornea and conjunctiva, leading to significant visual impairment or loss. Management includes immediate and thorough irrigation, followed by intensive medical therapy to reduce inflammation, prevent infection, and promote healing. Advanced treatments such as amniotic membrane transplantation and limbal stem cell transplantation may be necessary to restore ocular surface integrity [10].

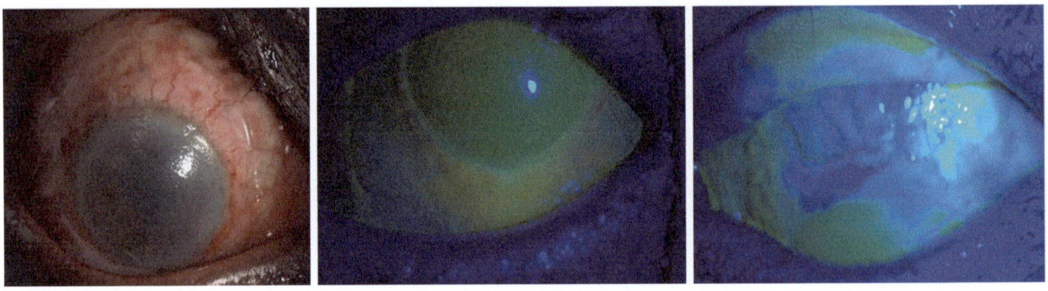

Diffuse illumination slit lamp images of a patient depicting

- Moderate–severe grade of chemical injury involving 100% corneal and conjunctival epithelial defects and complete involvement of limbus; no evidence of ischemia exposure
- EPIX classification of acute chemical injury: unilateral grade 6: E6-P0/I0/X0 [L6, C4, K2, T2]
- E—epithelial defect (L—limbal, C—conjunctival, K—Corneal, T—tarsal)
- P—intraocular pressure
- I—ischemia
- X—exposure

3.4.3 Limbal and Scleral Ischemia

Limbal and scleral ischemia following a lime injury can result in severe ocular surface damage, potentially leading to permanent vision loss. Immediate and aggressive treatment is required, including debridement of necrotic tissue, anti-inflammatory therapy, and surgical interventions such as amniotic membrane transplantation or limbal stem cell transplantation to restore vascularity and promote healing [11].

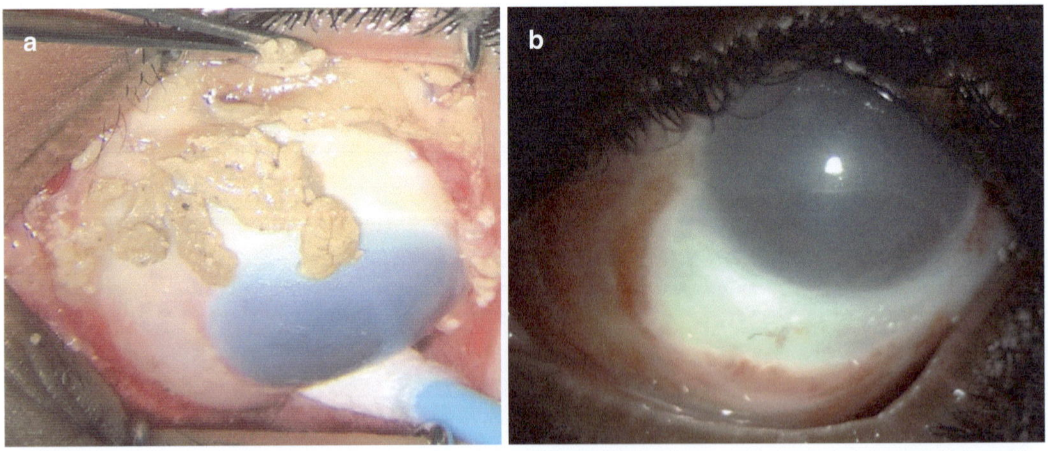

Diffuse illumination slit lamp image of a patient depicting: (**a**) Retained lime in the superior fornix with underlying scleral ischemia in a child following injury with chuna "lime". (**b**) Scleral ischemia involving almost 5 clock hours of inferior limbus in a patient following acid injury

3.5 Stevens-Johnson Syndrome

3.5.1 Partial Limbal Stem Cell Deficiency

Stevens-Johnson syndrome (SJS) is a severe mucocutaneous disorder often triggered by medications or infections. Ocular involvement includes severe conjunctivitis, corneal ulcers, and symblepharon formation. Management focuses on acute care with systemic immunosuppression and long-term ocular surface rehabilitation, including amniotic membrane transplantation and limbal stem cell transplantation [13].

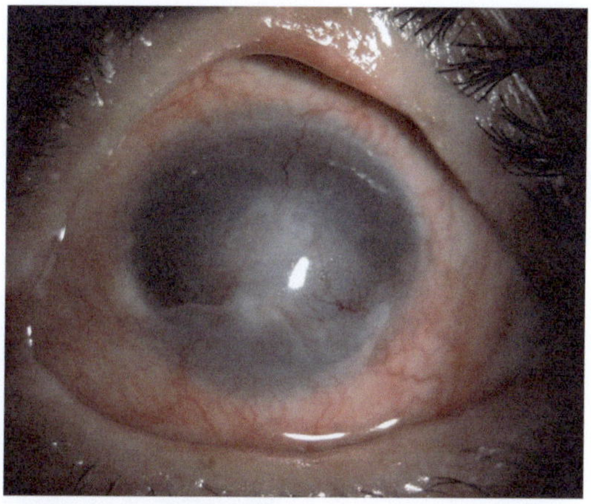

Diffuse illumination slit lamp image of a patient depicting conjunctival congestion, partial LSCD, and central corneal scar with superficial vascularization in a patient with Stevens-Johnson syndrome

3.5.2 Total Limbal Stem Cell Deficiency

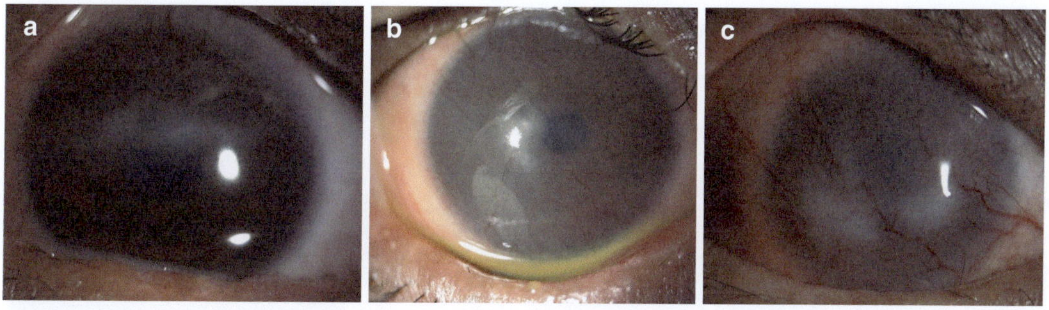

Diffuse illumination slit lamp image of a patient depicting: (**a**) Partial sectoral limbal stem cell deficiency sparing the inferior cornea in a patient with Stevens-Johnson syndrome. (**b**) Diffuse partial limbal stem cell deficiency sparing the central cornea in a patient with Stevens-Johnson syndrome. (**c**) Total limbal stem cell deficiency in a patient with Stevens-Johnson syndrome

3.5.3 Inclusion Cyst

Stevens-Johnson syndrome (SJS) can lead to the formation of inclusion cysts on the ocular surface, resulting from the severe inflammatory response and subsequent healing process. These cysts may cause discomfort and visual disturbance, often requiring surgical excision to restore normal ocular surface anatomy and function [14].

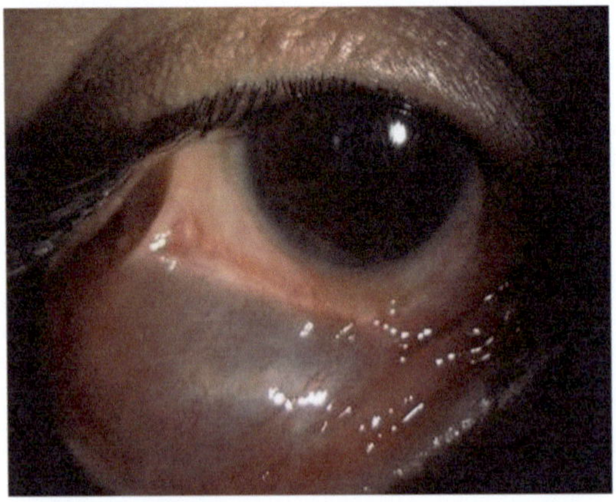

Diffuse illumination slit lamp image of a patient depicting conjunctival inclusion cyst in the lower tarsal conjunctiva and fornix in a patient with Stevens-Johnson syndrome

3.5.4 Lid Margin Keratinization

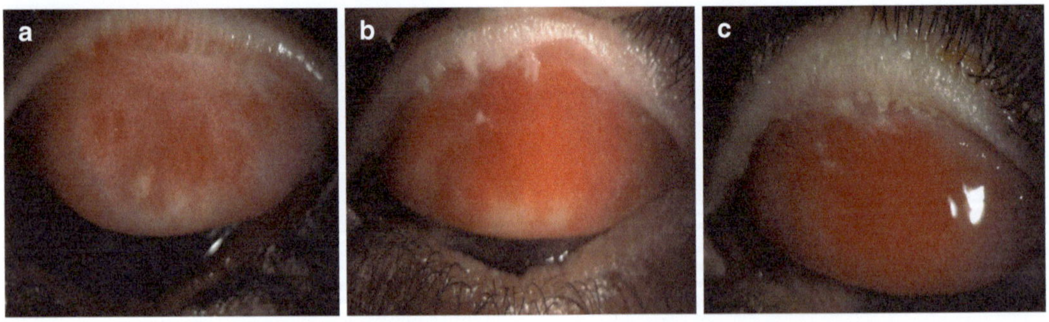

Diffuse illumination slit lamp image of the patient with Stevens-Johnson Syndrome depicting: (**a**) Grade 1 lid margin keratinization: mild irregularity of the mucocutaneous junction. (**b**) Grade 2 lid margin keratinization: moderate irregularity of the mucocutaneous junction. (**c**) Grade 3 lid margin keratinization: severe irregularity of the mucocutaneous junction irregularity

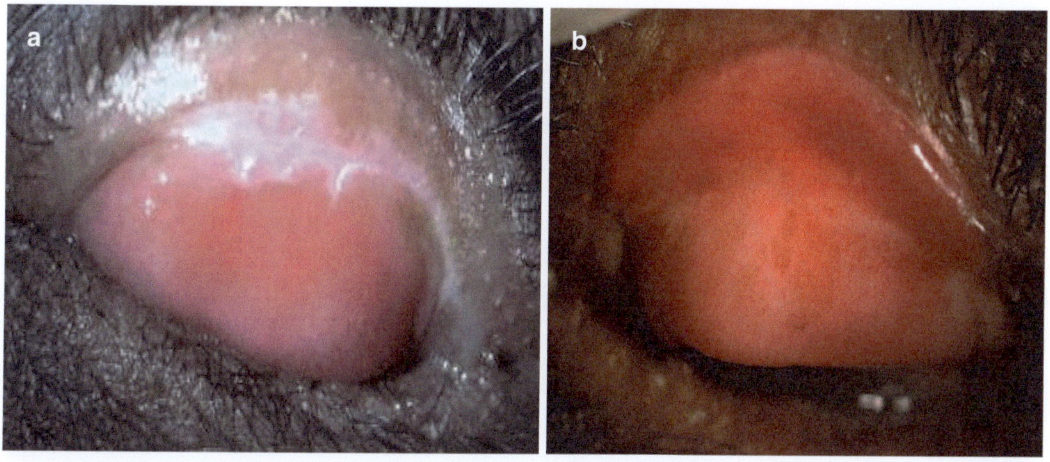

Diffuse illumination slit lamp image of a patient depicting: (**a**) Lid margin keratinization (LMK) causing blink-related microtrauma in a patient with Stevens-Johnson syndrome. (**b**) Excision of LMK, followed by mucous membrane graft harvested from the lower lip to reduce the same

3.5.5 Mucous Membrane Grafting

3.5.5.1 Mucous Membrane Grafts

Mucous membrane grafts, typically harvested from the oral mucosa, are used in reconstructive surgery of the ocular surface, particularly in severe conjunctival cicatrization cases. These grafts provide a stable epithelial surface and promote healing, improving ocular comfort and function [15].

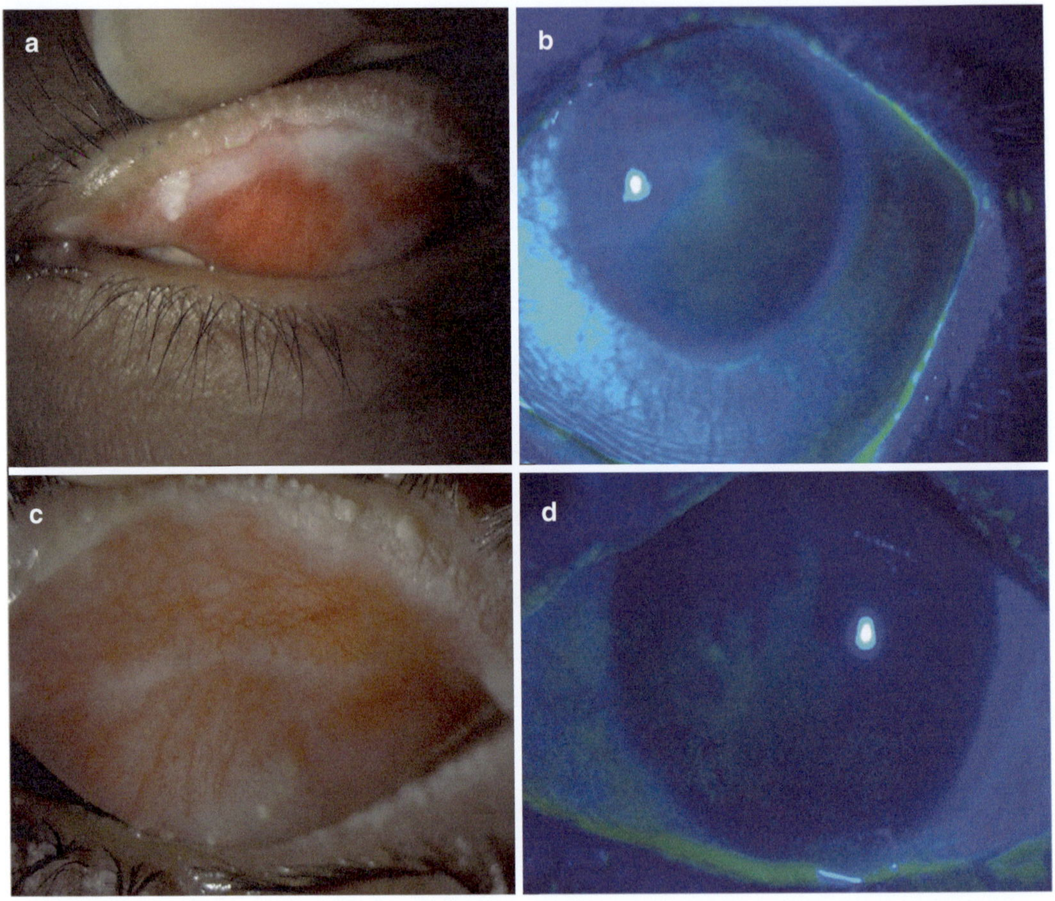

Diffuse illumination slit lamp image of a patient depicting: (**a**, **b**) Lid margin keratinization (LMK) causing blink-related microtrauma in a patient with Stevens-Johnson syndrome resulting in diffuse punctate keratitis. (**c**, **d**) Significant reduction in superficial punctate keratitis following excision of lid margin keratinization and mucous membrane graft 1 month following surgery

3.6 Vernal Keratoconjunctivitis

3.6.1 Limbal Papillae and Horner-Trantas Dots

Vernal keratoconjunctivitis (VKC) is a chronic allergic eye disease affecting primarily young males. It presents with intense itching, photophobia, and thick mucus discharge. Treatment includes topical antihistamines, mast cell stabilizers, and corticosteroids. In severe cases, immunosuppressants and surgical interventions may be necessary [16].

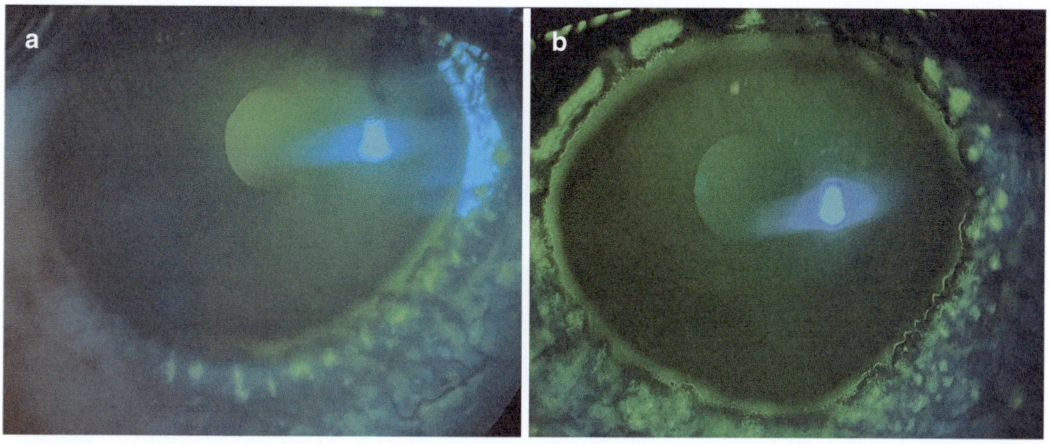

Diffuse illumination slit lamp image of a patient depicting (**a**) limbal papillae and (**b**) Horner-Trantas dots

3.6.2 Horner-Trantas Dots and Limbal Hypertrophy

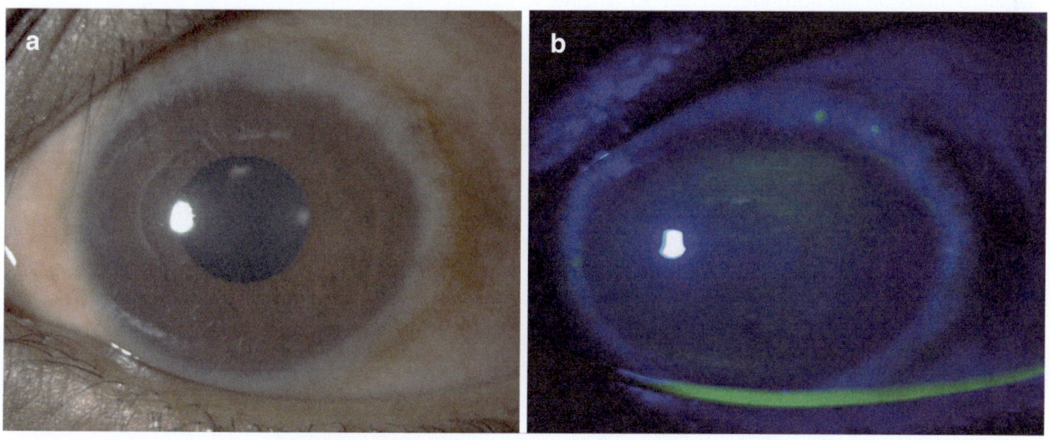

Diffuse illumination slit lamp image of a patient depicting: (**a**) Hypertrophied limbus with Horner-Trantas (HT) dots indicating limbal activity. (**b**) Fluorescein staining delineating the hypertrophied limbus and the HT

3.6.3 Shield Ulcer

Shield ulcers are large, superficial corneal epithelial defects associated with VKC. They result from chronic inflammation and mechanical trauma due to rubbing. Management includes anti-inflammatory treatments and therapeutic contact lenses to promote healing [17].

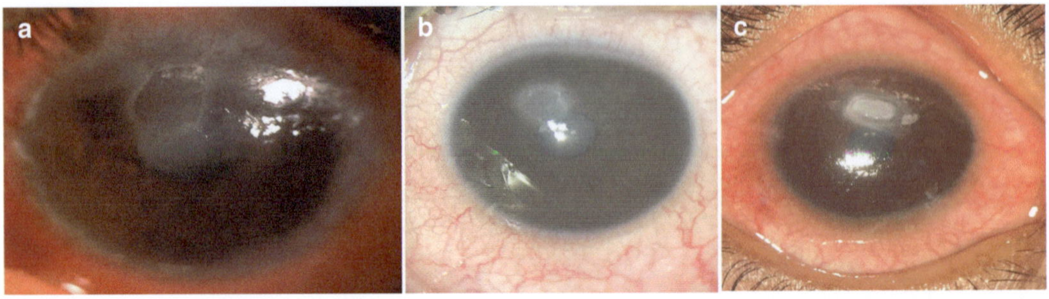

Diffuse illumination slit lamp image of a patient depicting: (**a**) Grade 1: Oval ulcer in the superior part of cornea with a relatively clear base in a patient with VKC in active disease state. (**b**) Grade 2: Oval ulcer in the superior part of cornea with minimal fibrin deposits over the base in a patient with VKC in active disease state. (**c**) Grade 3: Dense fibrin plaque deposited over the base of the ulcer in a patient with VKC in active disease state

3.6.4 Conjunctival Pigmentation

Vernal keratoconjunctivitis (VKC) can lead to conjunctival pigmentation, characterized by darkened areas on the conjunctiva due to chronic inflammation and immune responses. This pigmentation can be exacerbated by repeated episodes of inflammation and is often seen in conjunction with other ocular surface changes such as papillary hypertrophy and limbal thickening [18].

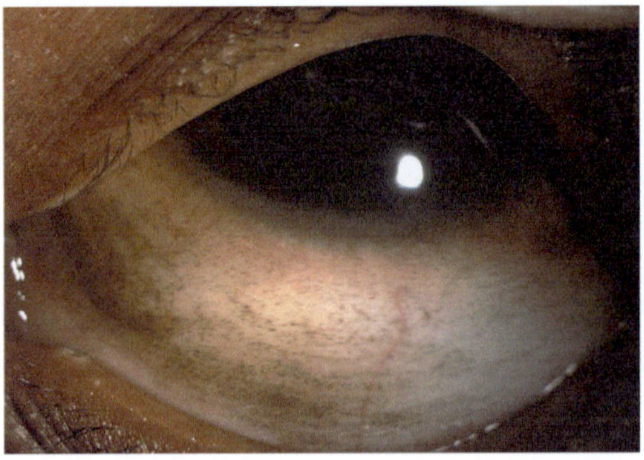

Diffuse illumination slit lamp image of a patient depicting diffuse conjunctival pigmentation in a patient with VKC

3.6.5 Papillary Reaction and Horner-Trantas Dots

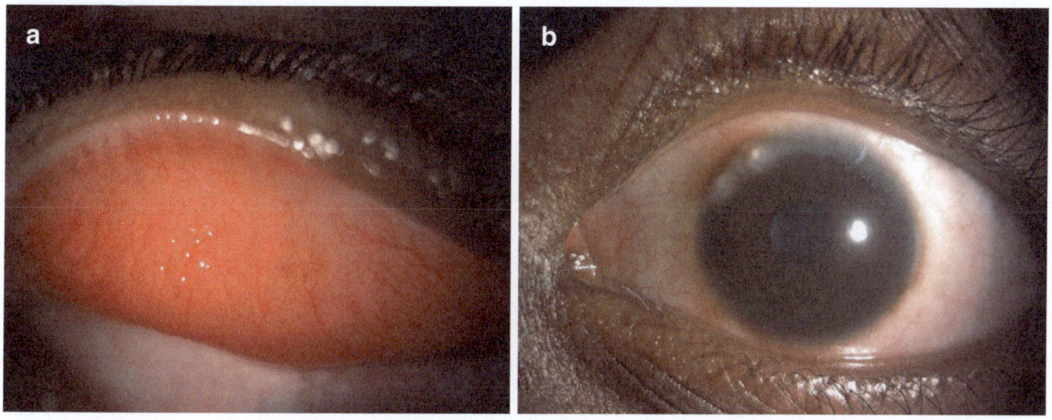

Diffuse illumination slit lamp image of a patient depicting signs of active vernal keratoconjunctivitis: (**a**) Tarsal papillary reaction. (**b**) Horner-Trantas dots with hypertrophied limbus

3.6.6 Tarsal Papillae

Vernal keratoconjunctivitis (VKC) often presents with large, cobblestone-like tarsal papillae on the upper eyelids. These hypertrophic papillae result from chronic inflammation and mechanical irritation, causing discomfort, itching, and potentially leading to corneal complications if left untreated [19].

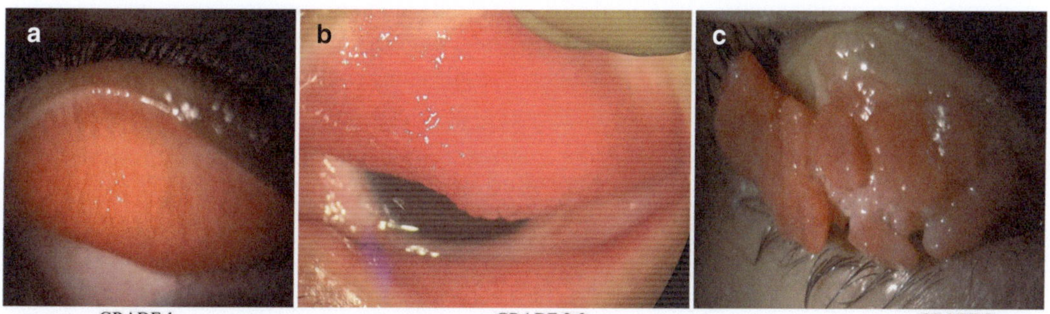

Diffuse illumination slit lamp image of a patient depicting papillary hyperplasia in the tarsal conjunctiva indicating an active VKC: (**a**) Grade 1: Size ranging from 0.1–0.2 mm. (**b**) Grade 2: size ranging from 0.3–0.9 mm. (**c**) Grade 3/cobblestone papillae: 1 mm and above

3.6.7 Mucous Membrane Grafting

Mucous membrane grafting in vernal keratoconjunctivitis (VKC) is utilized to manage severe conjunctival scarring and symblepharon formation. This surgical intervention helps restore the ocular surface integrity and function by providing a stable epithelial surface, reducing inflammation, and preventing further conjunctival fibrosis [20].

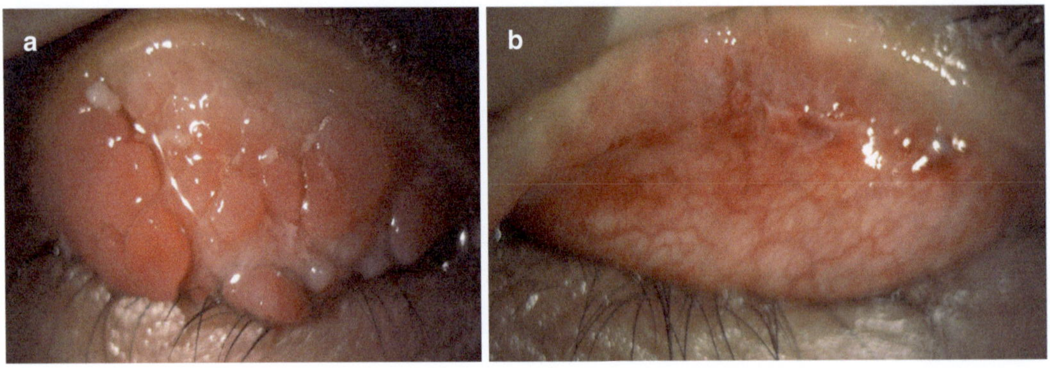

Diffuse illumination slit lamp image of a patient depicting: (**a**) Refractory giant cobblestone papillae causing recurrent shield ulcer in a 6-year-old child with severe vernal keratoconjunctivitis. (**b**) No recurrence of papillae along with a significant reduction in the frequency of episodes of VKC disease activity, 1 year following excision of papillae with mucous membrane grafting

3.6.8 Dense Fibrin Plaque

In vernal keratoconjunctivitis (VKC), dense fibrin plaques can form on the cornea due to chronic inflammation and persistent epithelial defects. These plaques contribute to severe discomfort and visual impairment, requiring intensive anti-inflammatory treatment and, in some cases, surgical debridement to restore clear vision and alleviate symptoms [16].

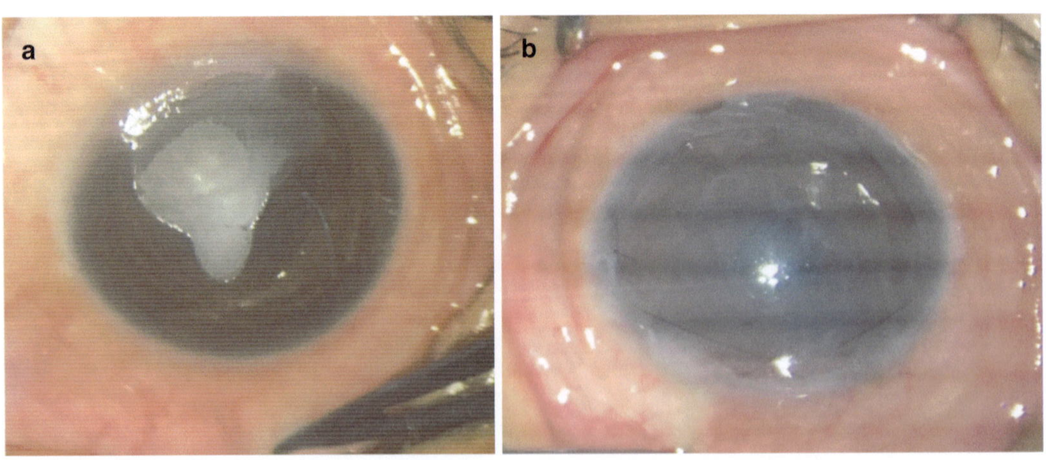

Diffuse illumination slit lamp image of a patient depicting: (**a**) Grade 3 shield ulcer with dense fibrin plaque at the base. (**b**) Superficial keratectomy along with perilimbal amniotic membrane transplant along with bandage contact lens placed to facilitate rapid epithelialization

3.7 Corneal Tattooing

Corneal tattooing is a cosmetic procedure to improve the appearance of corneal scars and opacities. It involves applying pigment to the corneal stroma to mask defects and enhance the eye's cosmetic appearance. This technique can also reduce glare and photophobia in patients with iris defects [21].

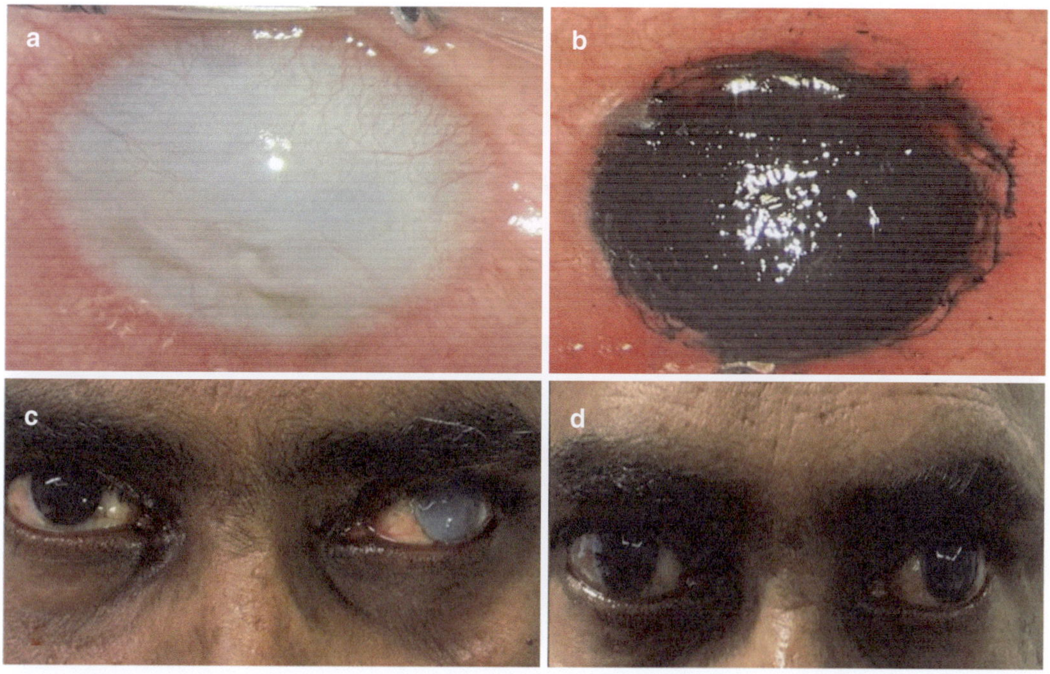

Diffuse illumination slit lamp image of a patient depicting: (**a**, **c**) Scarred cornea. (**b**, **d**) Post-corneal tattooing using the lamellar pocket technique

3.8 Ocular Cicatricial Pemphigoid

3.8.1 Conjunctival Fibrosis and Scarring

Ocular cicatricial pemphigoid (OCP) is a chronic autoimmune condition causing progressive conjunctival fibrosis and scarring. It leads to severe dry eye, symblepharon, and potential vision loss. Treatment involves systemic immunosuppression and surgical interventions to manage complications [22].

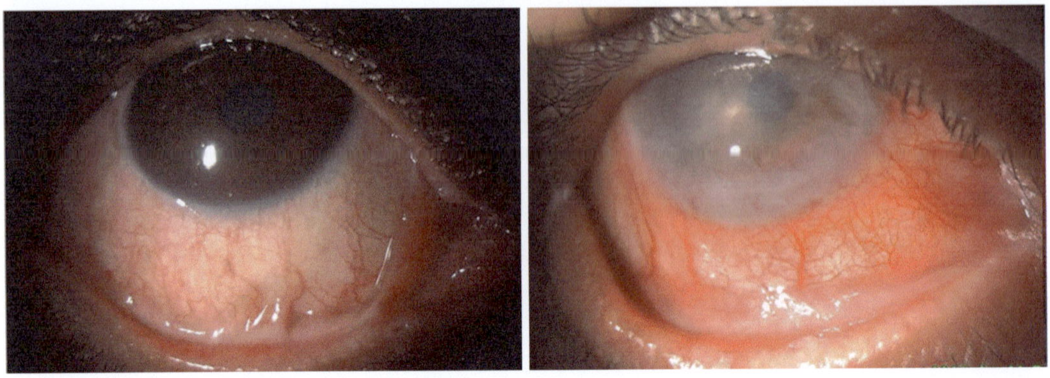

Diffuse illumination slit lamp image of a patient depicting early and diffuse forniceal shortening in OCP with inflamed ocular surface

3.8.2 Punctal Stenosis

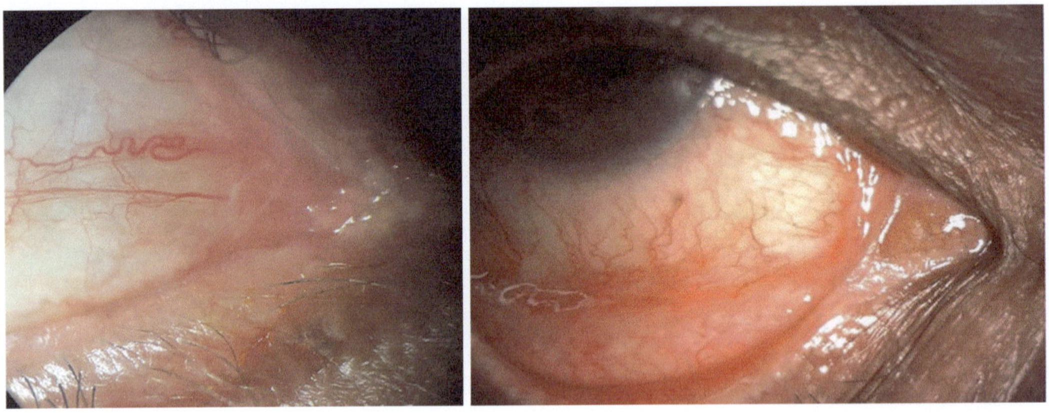

Diffuse illumination slit lamp image of a patient with ocular cicatricial pemphigoid depicting medial canthal keratinization with punctal stenosis

References

1. Sejpal K, Ali MH, Maddileti S, Basu S, Ramappa M, Kekunnaya R, et al. Cultivated limbal epithelial transplantation in children with ocular surface burns. JAMA Ophthalmol. 2013;131(6):731–6.
2. Shortt AJ, Secker GA, Notara MD, Limb GA, Khaw PT, Tuft SJ, Daniels JT. Transplantation of ex vivo cultured limbal epithelial stem cells: a review of techniques and clinical results. Surv Ophthalmol. 2007;52(5):483–502.
3. Dua HS, Azuara-Blanco A. Limbal stem cells of the corneal epithelium. Surv Ophthalmol. 2000;44(5):415–25.
4. Sangwan VS, Basu S, MacNeil S, Balasubramanian D. Simple limbal epithelial transplantation (SLET): a novel surgical technique for the treatment of unilateral limbal stem cell deficiency. Br J Ophthalmol. 2012;96(7):931–4.
5. Tsubota K, Satake Y, Kaido M, Shinozaki N, Shimmura S, Bissen-Miyajima H, et al. Treatment of severe ocular surface disorders with corneal epithelial stem-cell transplantation. N Engl J Med. 1999;340(22):1697–703.
6. Liu L, Wu J, Geng J, Yuan Z, Huang D. Geographical prevalence and risk factors for pterygium: a systematic review and meta-analysis. BMJ Open. 2013;3:11.
7. Mencucci R, Favuzza E, De Leucio R, Paladini I, Ambrosini S, Favuzza V. Clinical evaluation of persistent corneal epithelial defect treatment: a retrospective study. BMC Ophthalmol. 2018;18(1):192.
8. Dua HS, Said DG, Messmer EM, Rolando M, Benítez-Del-Castillo JM, Hossain PN, et al. Neurotrophic keratopathy. Prog Retin Eye Res. 2018;66:107–31.

9. Shanbhag SS, Shah S, Singh R, Donthineni PR, Basu S. Clinical outcomes of amniotic membrane transplantation and limbal stem cell transplantation in management of acute ocular chemical burns: a review of the literature. Br J Ophthalmol. 2020;104(2):182–7.
10. Singh P, Tyagi M, Kumar Y, Gupta KK, Sharma PD. Ocular chemical injuries and their management. Oman J Ophthalmol. 2013;6(2):83–6.
11. Kuckelkorn R, Schrage N, Keller G, Redbrake C, Reim M. Emergency treatment of chemical and thermal eye burns. Acta Ophthalmol Scand. 2002;80(1):4–10.
12. Aldave AJ, Sangwan VS, Basu S. The Boston keratoprosthesis: a review with an Indian perspective. Indian J Ophthalmol. 2020;68(4):558–64.
13. Kohanim S, Palioura S, Saeed HN, Akpek EK, Amescua G, Basu S, et al. Stevens-Johnson syndrome/toxic epidermal necrolysis—a comprehensive review and guide to therapy. I. Systemic disease. Ocul Surf. 2016;14(1):2–19.
14. Lee HY, Wee WR, Lee JH, Kim MK. Stevens-Johnson syndrome and toxic epidermal necrolysis: clinical outcomes of ocular complications. Cornea. 2017;36(4):408–13.
15. Tsubota K, Satake Y, Kaido M, Shimazaki J, Shinozaki N, Bissen-Miyajima H, et al. Surgical reconstruction of the ocular surface in advanced ocular cicatricial pemphigoid and Stevens-Johnson syndrome. Am J Ophthalmol. 1996;122(1):38–52.
16. Bonini S, Coassin M, Aronni S, Lambiase A. Vernal keratoconjunctivitis. Eye (Lond). 2004;18(4):345–51.
17. Bonini S, Lambiase A, Marchi S, Pasqualetti P, Zuccaro O, Rama P. Vernal keratoconjunctivitis revisited: a case series of 195 patients with long-term follow-up. Ophthalmology. 2000;107(6):1157–63.
18. Tabbara KF, al-Kharashi SA. Vernal keratoconjunctivitis in Saudi Arabia: clinical and immunological aspects. Acta Ophthalmol Scand. 1999;77(5):557–61.
19. Leonardi A, Secchi AG. Vernal keratoconjunctivitis. Int Ophthalmol Clin. 2003;43(1):41–58.
20. Dua HS, Azuara-Blanco A. Allo-limbal transplantation in patients with limbal stem cell deficiency. Br J Ophthalmol. 1999;83(4):414–9.
21. Alio JL, Sirerol B, Walewska-Szafran A, Miranda M, Montés-Micó R. Corneal tattooing (keratopigmentation) for the management of eye aesthetic disorders and iris defects. Br J Ophthalmol. 2010;94(2):245–9.
22. Foster CS, Sainz de la Maza M. Ocular cicatricial pemphigoid review. Curr Opin Allergy Clin Immunol. 2004;4(5):435–9.

4 Congenital Anomalies of the Cornea and Sclera

Shweta Agarwal, Bhaskar Srinivasan, and Geetha Iyer

4.1 Introduction

Congenital anomalies of the cornea and sclera are diverse conditions present at birth that can significantly impact ocular health and vision. These anomalies can result from genetic mutations, developmental disturbances, or environmental factors affecting the developing eye. Understanding these conditions is crucial for early diagnosis, appropriate management, and genetic counseling. This chapter covers several key congenital anomalies, including secondary abnormalities affecting the infant cornea, limbal dermoid, congenital staphyloma, congenital glaucoma, congenital sclerocornea, birth trauma, metabolic disorders, posterior embryotoxon, aniridia, Axenfeld-Rieger anomaly, and iridocorneal endothelial (ICE) syndrome.

4.2 Limbal Dermoid

4.2.1 Grade 1 Limbal Dermoid

Limbal dermoids are benign congenital growths containing ectodermal elements, such as hair follicles and sebaceous glands. They typically present as whitish, elevated masses at the corneolimbal junction and can cause astigmatism or visual obstruction. Surgical excision is often required for cosmetic and functional reasons [1].

S. Agarwal (✉) · B. Srinivasan · G. Iyer
CJ Shah Cornea Services, Medical Research Foundation, Sankara Nethralaya, Chennai, Tamil Nadu, India

B. Gurnani, K. Kaur (eds.), *Atlas of Cornea*, https://doi.org/10.1007/978-981-96-0013-7_4

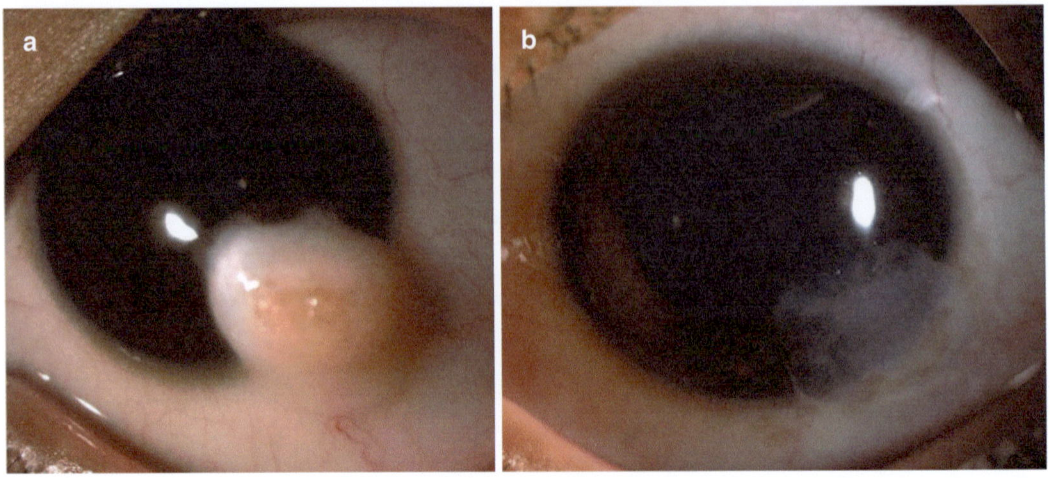

Diffuse illumination slit lamp image of a patient depicting: (**a**) Grade 1 limbal/epibulbar dermoid in a 6-year-old child causing significant astigmatism. (**b**) Underwent excision with amniotic membrane graft followed by glasses for visual rehabilitation

4.2.2 Grade 2 Limbal/Epibulbar Dermoid

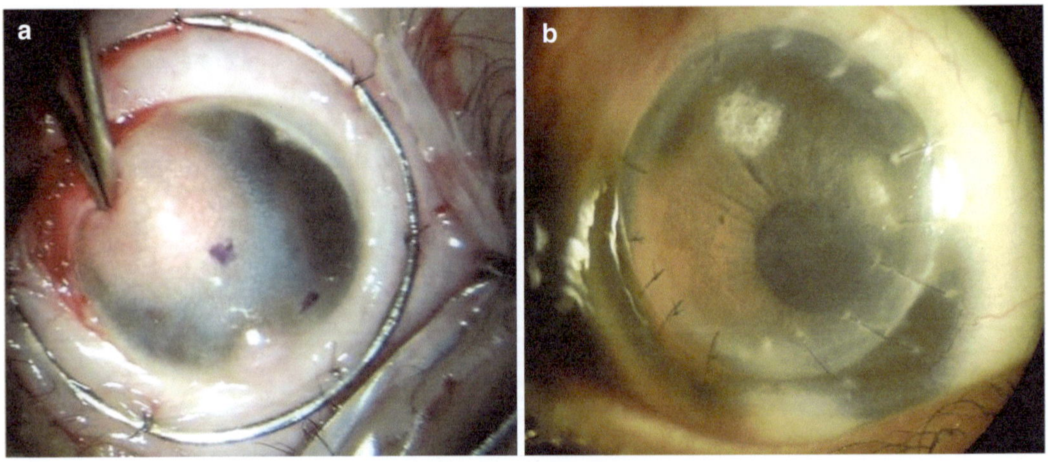

Diffuse illumination slit lamp image of a patient depicting: (**a**) Grade 2 limbal/epibulbar dermoid in a 7-year-old child causing amblyopia. (**b**) Underwent deep anterior lamellar keratoplasty to clear the visual axis followed by glasses and amblyopia therapy for visual rehabilitation

4.2.3 Penetrating Keratoplasty in Limbal Dermoid

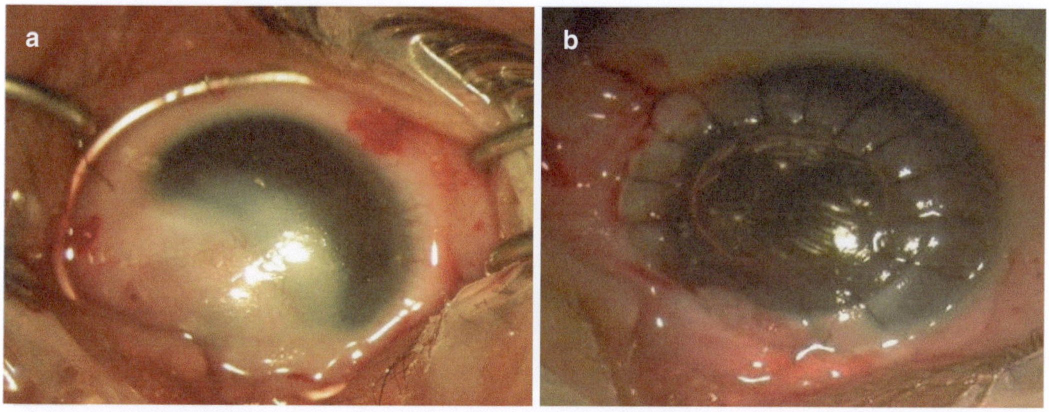

Diffuse illumination slit lamp image of a patient depicting: (**a**) Grade 2 limbal/epibulbar dermoid in a 4-year-old child causing amblyopia. (**b**) Underwent penetrating keratoplasty to clear the visual axis followed by glasses and amblyopia therapy for visual rehabilitation

4.2.4 Congenital Anterior Staphyloma

Congenital staphyloma is a protrusion of uveal tissue through a weak point in the cornea or sclera, present at birth. It can lead to significant visual impairment and requires prompt surgical intervention to prevent further ocular complications [2].

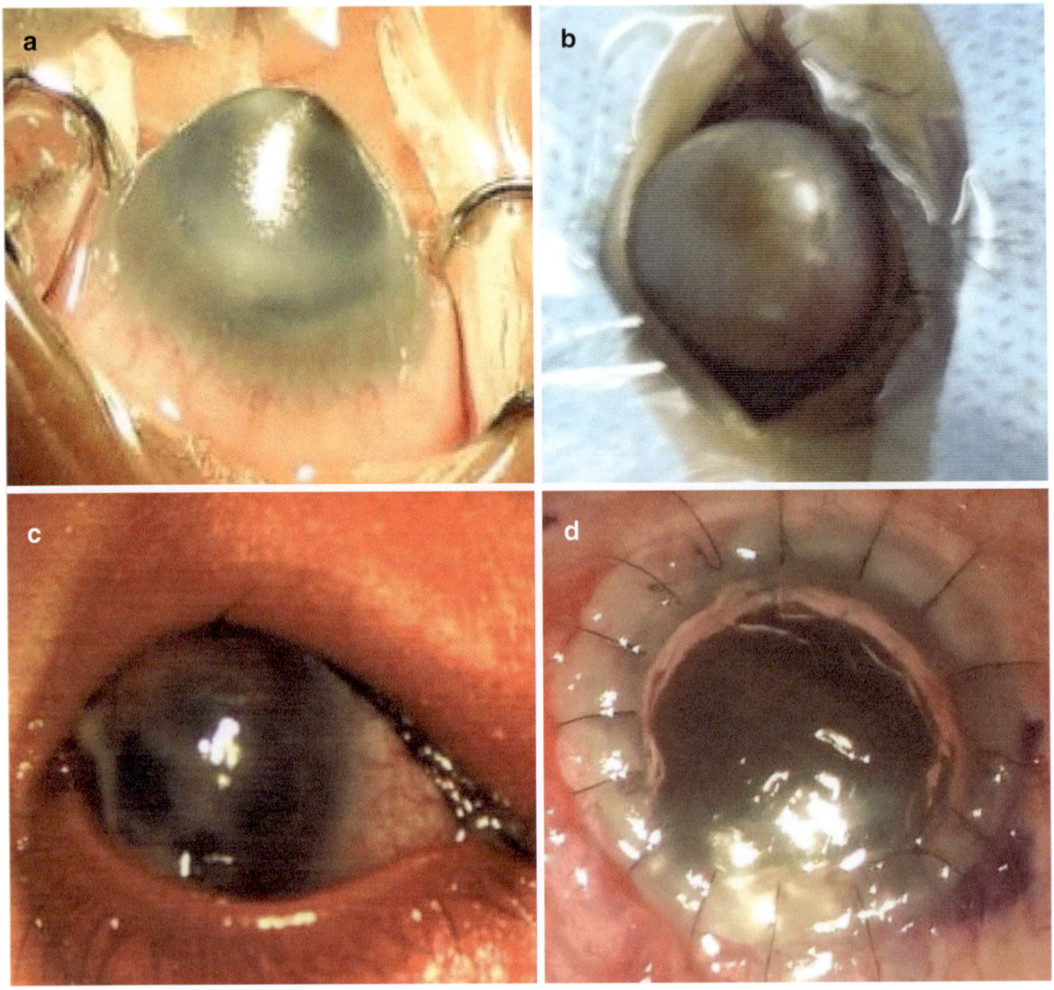

Diffuse illumination slit lamp image of a patient depicting: (**a**, **b**) Congenital anterior staphyloma. (**c**) Congenital anterior staphyloma in a 2-year-old boy. (**d**) Underwent limbal sparing penetrating keratoplasty with lensectomy maintaining 6 m finger counting vision for 3 years

4.3 Congenital Sclerocornea

4.3.1 Partial and Total Sclerocornea

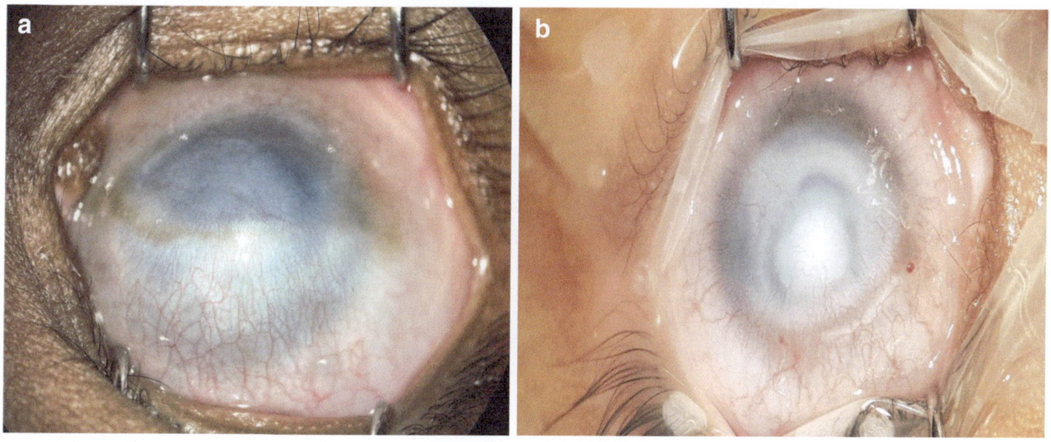

Diffuse illumination slit lamp image of a patient depicting: (**a**) Partial sclerocornea with corneal scarring. (**b**) Total sclerocornea with central thinning

4.3.2 Penetrating Keratoplasty in Congenital Sclerocornea

Congenital sclerocornea is a developmental anomaly where the cornea is opaque and resembles scleral tissue. It is often associated with other ocular and systemic anomalies. Management focuses on addressing associated visual impairments and ensuring appropriate visual development [3].

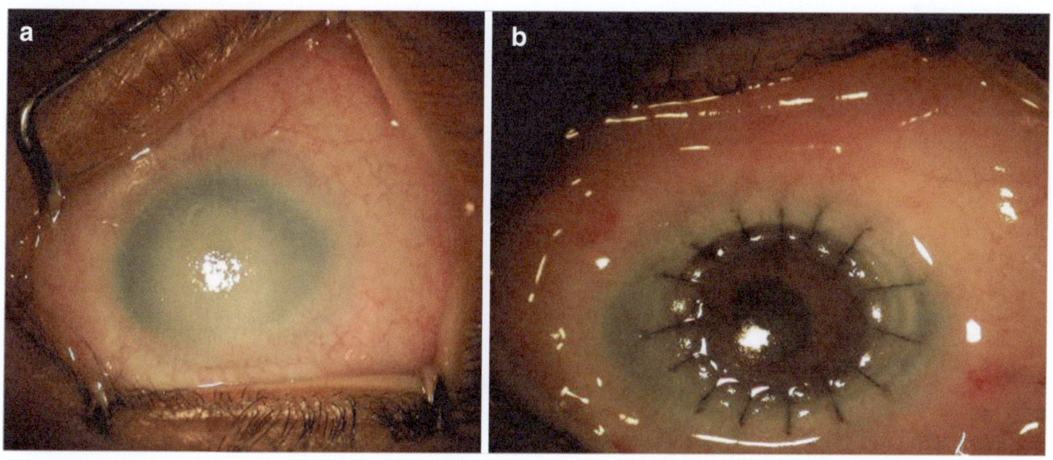

Diffuse illumination slit lamp image of a patient depicting: (**a**) Sclerization of the corneal surface with total corneal scarring with total limbal stem cell deficiency. (**b**) Post-optical penetrating keratoplasty in the same patient

4.3.3 Posterior Embryotoxon

Posterior embryotoxon is a congenital anomaly characterized by a prominent Schwalbe's line, visible as a white line on the posterior cornea. While often asymptomatic, it can be associated with other anterior segment dysgenesis conditions, necessitating further evaluation [4].

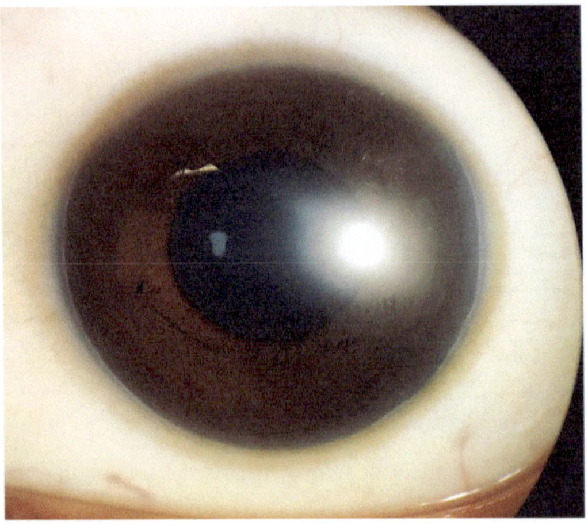

Diffuse slit lamp picture showing an anteriorly displaced Schwalbe line

4.3.4 Limbal Sparing Penetrating Keratoplasty with Allo-SLET

Limbal sparing penetrating keratoplasty combined with allo-SLET (allogeneic simple limbal epithelial transplantation) is an advanced surgical technique used to treat severe corneal disease with limbal stem cell deficiency. This approach preserves the limbal stem cells while replacing the damaged cornea, promoting better graft survival and ocular surface restoration [5].

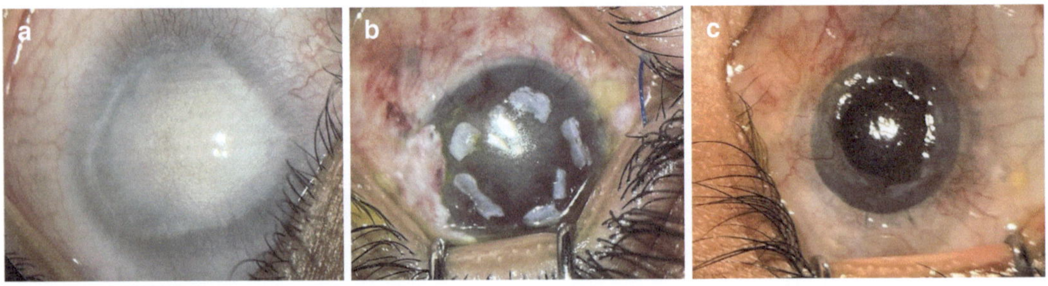

Diffuse illumination slit lamp image of a patient depicting: (**a**) Total sclerocornea with superficial vascularization. (**b**) Allo-simple limbal epithelial transplant in the same patient. (**c**) Limbal sparing penetrating keratoplasty after allo-simple limbal epithelial transplant

4.3.5 Aniridia

Aniridia is a rare congenital condition marked by the partial or complete absence of the iris, leading to significant visual impairment and associated anomalies such as foveal hypoplasia and nystagmus. Management involves optical correction and monitoring for glaucoma and other complications [6].

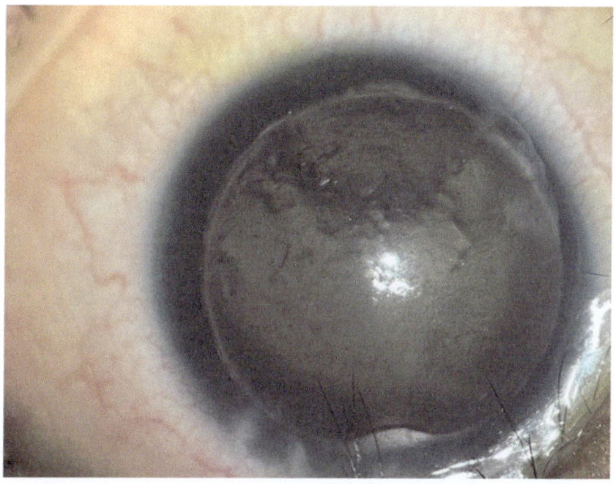

Diffuse illumination slit lamp image of a patient depicting congenital aniridia in a 5-year-old child

4.3.6 Axenfeld–Rieger Anomaly

Axenfeld–Rieger anomaly comprises a spectrum of anterior segment dysgenesis disorders, including abnormalities of the iris, cornea, and anterior chamber angle. It is associated with an increased risk of glaucoma and requires regular monitoring and management to preserve vision [4, 7].

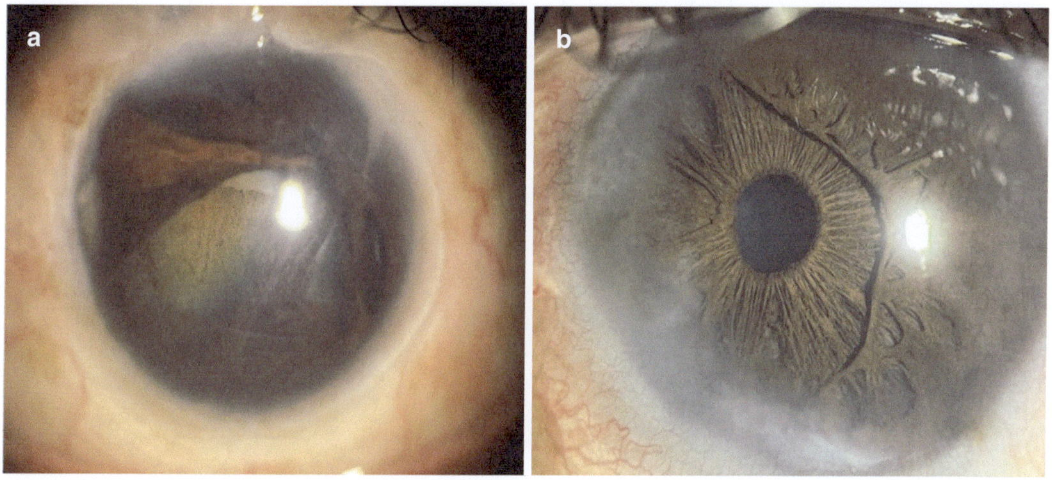

Diffuse slit lamp image of a patient with Axenfeld–Rieger anomaly depicting: (**a**) Limbal stem cell deficiency, correctopia, and polycoria. (**b**) Nasal sclerocornea with ectopic pupil

4.3.7 Iridocorneal Endothelial (ICE) Syndrome

ICE syndrome is a group of conditions characterized by abnormal corneal endothelial cells that migrate onto the iris and anterior chamber angle, leading to corneal edema, iris abnormalities, and secondary glaucoma. Management focuses on controlling intraocular pressure and addressing corneal edema [8].

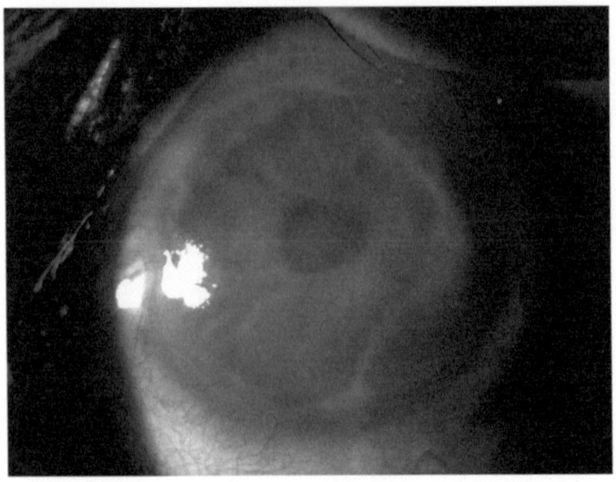

Diffuse illumination slit lamp image of a patient depicting corneal decompensation with iridocorneal endothelial syndrome (ICE)

References

1. Gonnering RS, Sonneland PR. Surgical management of limbal dermoids. Ophthalmology. 1985;92(5):619–23.
2. Khaw PT, Elkington AR. Congenital anterior staphyloma: management and visual prognosis. Br J Ophthalmol. 1992;76(6):351–3.
3. Segev F, Jaouni T, Schwartz M, Schwinger E, Rosenmann A. Sclerocornea and congenital coronary cataract in an inbred Bedouin kindred: possible linkage to the gene for beta-1,3-galactosyltransferase-like. Am J Hum Genet. 2000;67(6):1529–35.
4. Shields MB, Buckley E, Klintworth GK, Thresher R. Axenfeld-Rieger syndrome. A spectrum of developmental disorders. Surv Ophthalmol. 1985;29(6):387–409.
5. Basu S, Sureka SP, Shanbhag SS, Kethiri AR, Singh V. Simple limbal epithelial transplantation: long-term clinical outcomes in 125 cases of unilateral chronic ocular surface burns. Ophthalmology. 2016;123(5):1000–10.
6. Nelson LB, Spaeth GL, Nowinski TS, Margo CE, Jackson L. Aniridia. A review. Surv Ophthalmol. 1984;28(6):621–42.
7. Shields MB. Axenfeld-Rieger syndrome: a theory of mechanism and distinctions from the iridocorneal endothelial syndrome. Trans Am Ophthalmol Soc. 1983;81:736–84.
8. Shields MB. Iridocorneal endothelial syndrome: a specter of essential iris atrophy, Chandler's syndrome, and Cogan-Reese syndrome. Surv Ophthalmol. 1979;24(6):415–9.

Degenerations and Depositions

5

Aditi Parab, Josephine Christy S., Bharat Gurnani, and Kirandeep Kaur

5.1 Introduction

Ocular surface degenerations and depositions represent a group of conditions characterized by the accumulation of various materials within the ocular tissues, leading to structural and functional changes. These conditions can be congenital, acquired, or associated with systemic diseases, and they often impact the cornea and conjunctiva. This chapter provides an overview of several key degenerations and depositions, including conjunctival concretions, crocodile shagreen, arcus senilis, Salzmann's nodular degeneration, pterygium, conjunctival inclusion cyst, drug-induced corneal deposits, cornea verticillata, climatic droplet keratopathy, superficial punctate keratitis, subepithelial keratitis, desquamated corneal epithelium, lipid keratopathy, conjunctival cyst, and guttae.

A. Parab · J. Christy S. (✉)
Cornea and Refractive Services, Aravind Eye Hospital and Post Graduate Institute of Ophthalmology, Pondicherry, India

B. Gurnani
Department of Cataract, Cornea, Trauma, External Diseases, Ocular Surface and Refractive Services, Gomabai Netralaya and Research Centre, Neemuch, Madhya Pradesh, India

K. Kaur
Department of Cataract, Pediatric Ophthalmology and Strabismus, Gomabai Netralaya and Research Centre, Neemuch, Madhya Pradesh, India

5.1.1 Conjunctival Concretions

Conjunctival concretions are small, yellow-white deposits composed of epithelial debris and mucin located beneath the conjunctival epithelium. They are often asymptomatic but can cause irritation if they erode through the surface. Treatment is usually unnecessary unless symptomatic, in which case removal with a needle can be performed [1].

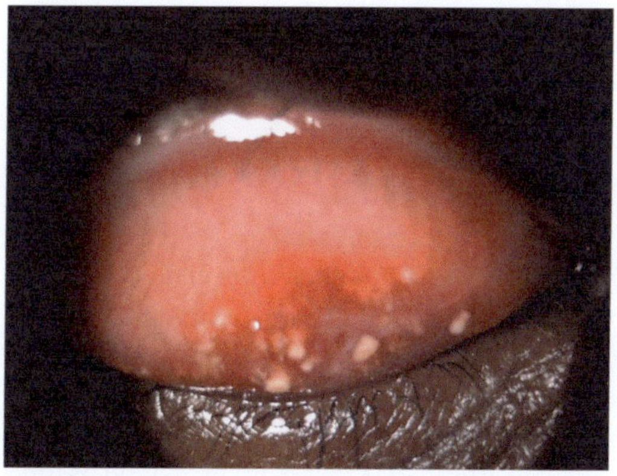

Figure illustrating conjunctival concretions which are small yellow-white lesions on palpebral conjunctiva consisting of degenerating epithelial cells and proteinaceous secretions

B. Gurnani, K. Kaur (eds.), *Atlas of Cornea*, https://doi.org/10.1007/978-981-96-0013-7_5

5.1.2 Crocodile Shagreen

Crocodile shagreen is characterized by polygonal, grayish-white opacities in the corneal stroma, typically found in the anterior or posterior cornea. It is generally benign and asymptomatic, often discovered incidentally during an eye examination. No treatment is required for this condition [2].

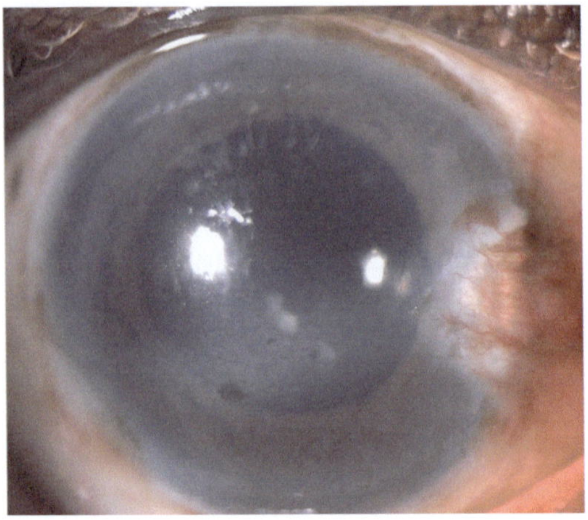

Figure depicting crocodile shagreen classically appearing as a bilateral localized area of polygonal opacities within the central posterior corneal stroma

5.1.3 Arcus Senilis

Arcus senilis is a common age-related condition where a white or grayish ring forms at the periphery of the cornea due to lipid deposition. It is usually bilateral and does not affect vision. Arcus senilis can also be seen in younger individuals with hyperlipidemia, warranting a lipid profile assessment in such cases [3].

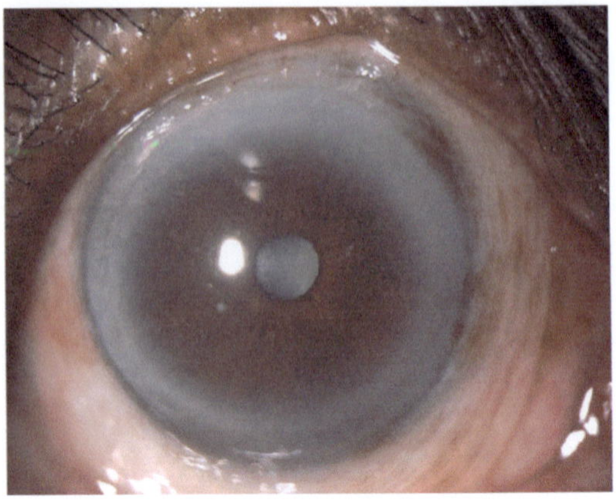

Figure showing dense arcus senilis appearing as a gray or white ring on the outer region of cornea due to lipid deposition

5.1.4 Salzmann's Nodular Degeneration

Salzmann's nodular degeneration involves the development of bluish-white nodules on the corneal surface, often secondary to chronic keratitis. It can cause visual impairment due to irregular astigmatism. Management includes lubricants, and in severe cases, surgical removal of the nodules [4].

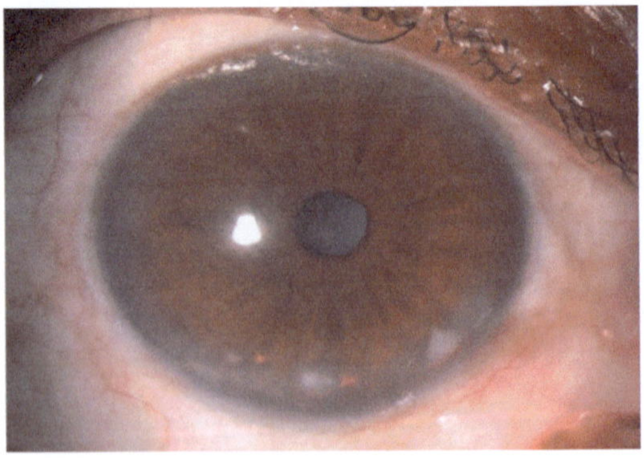

Figure depicting grayish white to bluish nodules anterior to Bowman's layer in the corneal periphery suggestive of Salzmann's nodular degeneration

5.1.5 Pterygium

Pterygium is a fibrovascular growth extending from the conjunctiva onto the cornea, associated with UV exposure and chronic irritation. It can lead to astigmatism and visual impairment if it encroaches on the visual axis. Treatment involves surgical excision, often combined with conjunctival autografting or amniotic membrane transplantation to reduce recurrence [5].

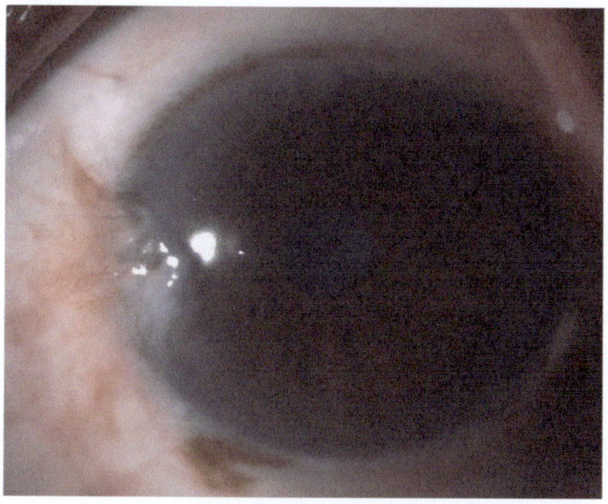

Figure illustrating pterygium, a wing-shaped degenerative ocular surface lesion originating from the limbal conjunctiva within the palpebral fissure

5.1.6 Conjunctival Inclusion Cyst

Conjunctival inclusion cysts are fluid-filled sacs on the conjunctiva, often resulting from trauma or surgery. They are generally benign and asymptomatic but can be excised if they cause discomfort or cosmetic concerns [6].

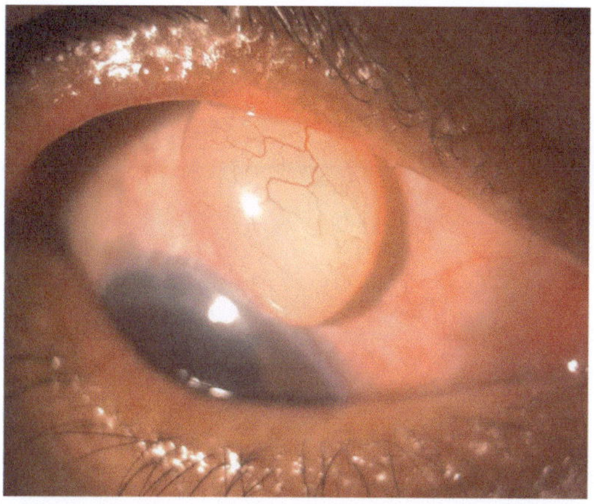

Figure illustrating conjunctival inclusion cyst which is a thin-walled benign cystic lesion containing serous fluid

5.1.7 Drug-Induced Corneal Deposits

Certain medications can lead to corneal deposits, such as amiodarone-induced vortex keratopathy and chloroquine deposits. These deposits can cause visual disturbances depending on their location and density. Discontinuation or adjustment of the offending drug often leads to resolution [7, 8].

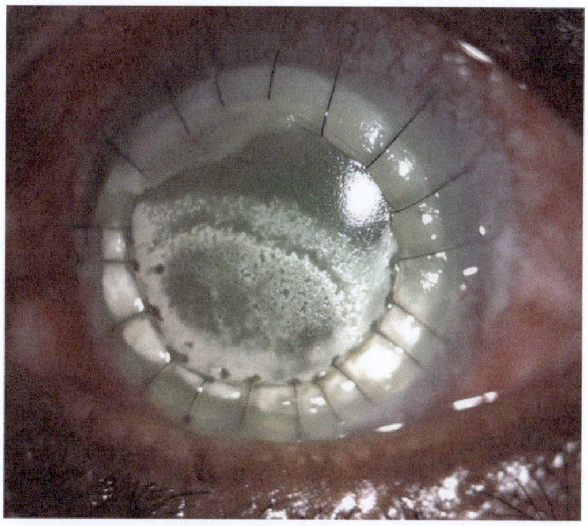

Figure illustrating the whitish epithelial deposits involving the visual axis over the graft post-penetrating keratoplasty

5.1.8 Drug-Induced Corneal Deposits

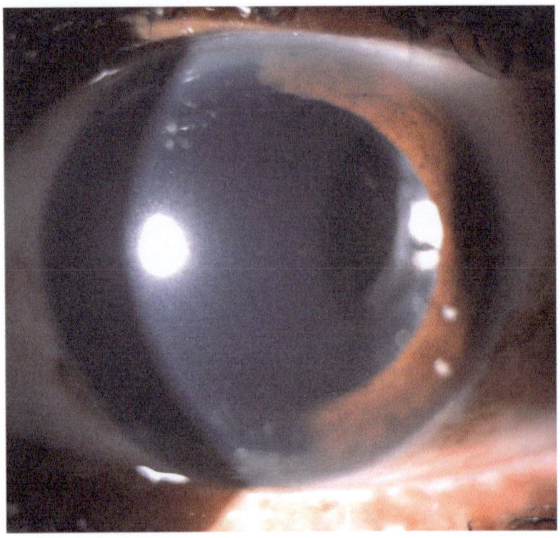

Figure showing tiny pigmented deposits over the cornea due to the consumption of the drug sodium valproate

5.1.9 Cornea Verticillata

Cornea verticillata, also known as vortex keratopathy, presents as whorl-like epithelial deposits typically induced by medications like amiodarone. It is usually asymptomatic and does not require treatment unless associated with visual symptoms [9].

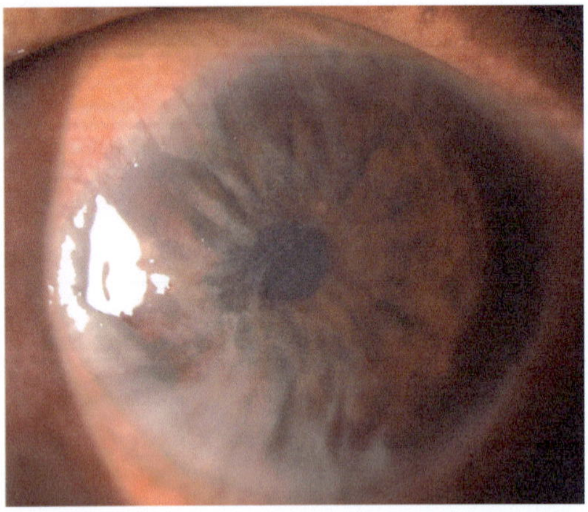

Figure illustrating vortex keratopathy characterized by the classical whorl-like pattern of grayish opacities in the corneal epithelium

5.1.10 Climatic Droplet Keratopathy

Climatic droplet keratopathy is characterized by the deposition of translucent droplets in the corneal stroma, commonly seen in older individuals living in tropical climates. It can cause visual impairment, and treatment includes UV protection and, in severe cases, keratectomy [10].

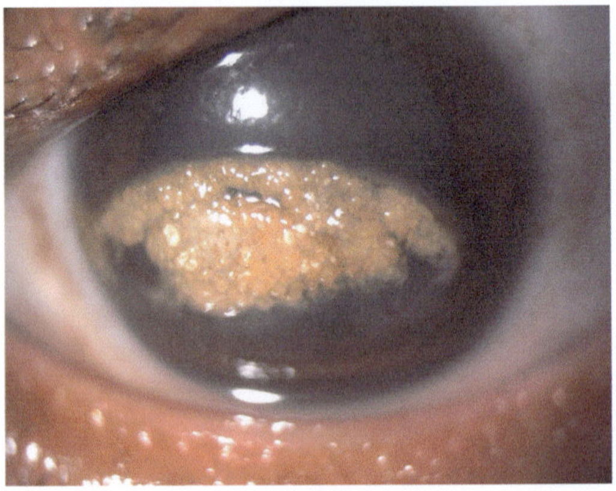

Figure illustrating homogeneous, translucent, golden yellow spherules or globules in the superficial stroma suggestive of climatic droplet keratopathy

5.1.11 Superficial Punctate Keratitis

Superficial punctate keratitis involves the presence of small, pinpoint epithelial erosions on the corneal surface, often due to dry eye, contact lens wear, or exposure to irritants. Management focuses on addressing the underlying cause and providing lubricating eye drops [11].

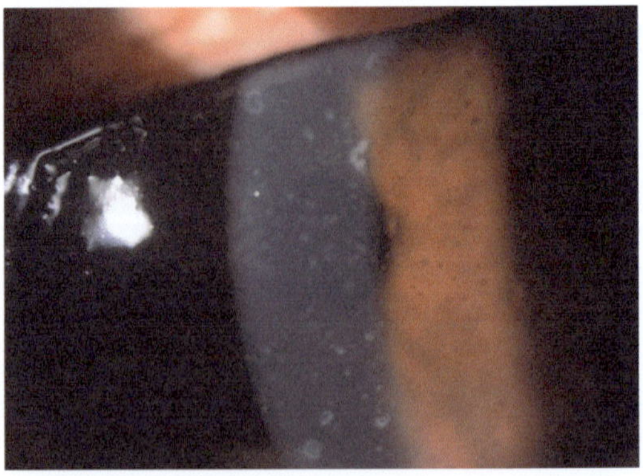

Figure illustrating superficial punctate keratitis characterized by fine, punctate corneal epithelial damage caused by diverse causes like herpes simplex virus, adenovirus, and microsporidium

5.1.12 Subepithelial Keratitis

Subepithelial keratitis presents with inflammatory infiltrates beneath the corneal epithelium, commonly seen in viral infections like adenoviral keratoconjunctivitis. It can cause decreased vision and photophobia. Treatment includes topical steroids and antiviral agents if necessary [12].

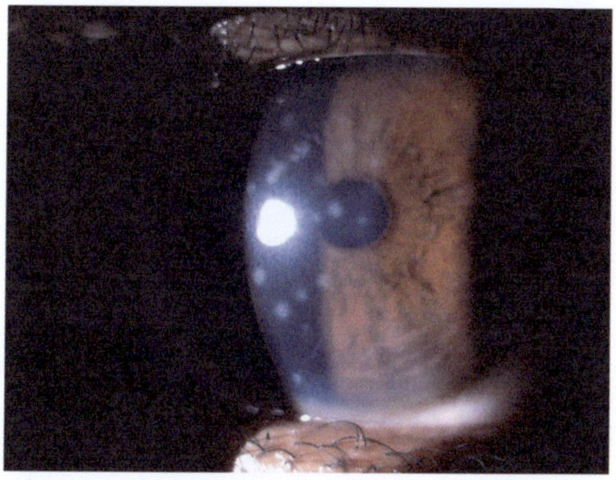

Digital slit image of a patient depicting multiple subepithelial infiltrates in a patient with adenoviral keratitis

5.1.13 Desquamated Corneal Epithelium

Desquamated corneal epithelium refers to the shedding of the corneal epithelial cells, often associated with underlying corneal dystrophies or trauma. Management includes lubrication, and in severe cases, bandage contact lenses or surgical intervention [13].

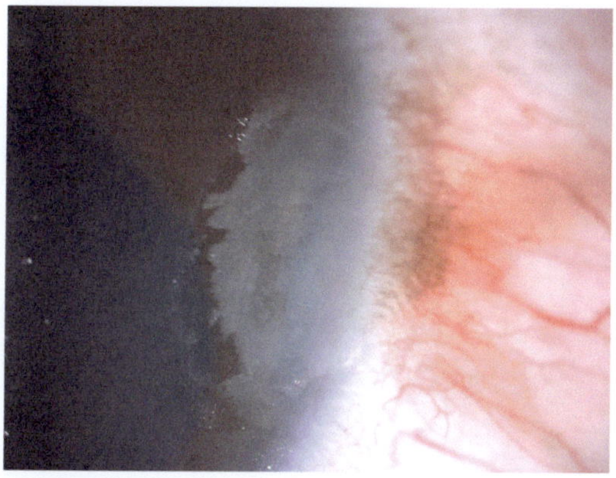

Diffuse illumination slit lamp image of a patient depicting desquamated corneal epithelium

5.1.14 Lipid Keratopathy

Lipid keratopathy involves the deposition of lipids in the cornea, usually following chronic inflammation or trauma. It appears as yellow-white deposits within the corneal stroma. Management focuses on treating the underlying cause and, in some cases, surgical intervention to remove the deposits [14].

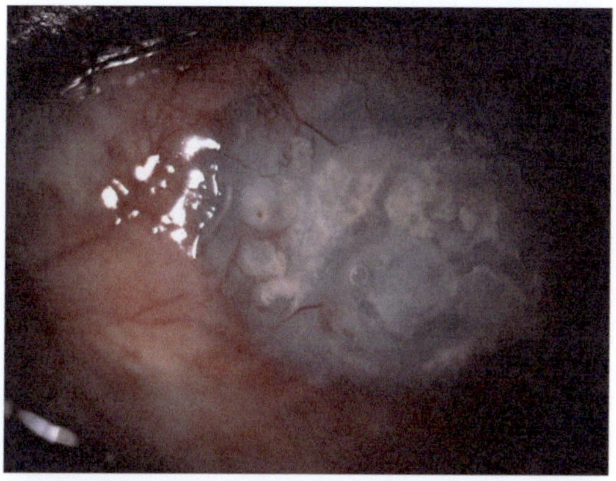

Digital diffuse illumination slit lamp image of a patient depicting lipid deposits in the cornea along with neovascularization in a patient with herpes simplex keratitis

5.1.15 Conjunctival Cyst

Conjunctival cysts are benign fluid-filled sacs on the conjunctiva that can result from inflammation, trauma, or surgery. They are typically asymptomatic but can be excised if they cause discomfort or cosmetic issues [15].

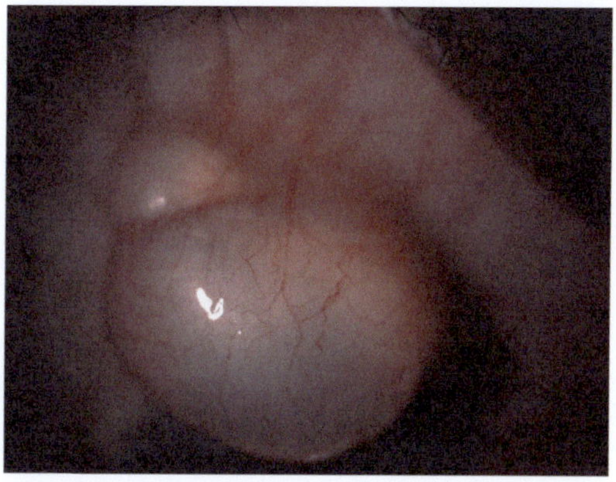

Diffuse illumination slit lamp image of a patient depicting conjunctival cyst with filled serous fluid

5.1.16 Guttae

Guttae are excrescences of the Descemet membrane seen in conditions like Fuchs' endothelial dystrophy. They appear as small, wart-like projections and can lead to corneal edema and visual impairment. Treatment includes managing corneal edema and, in advanced cases, endothelial keratoplasty [16].

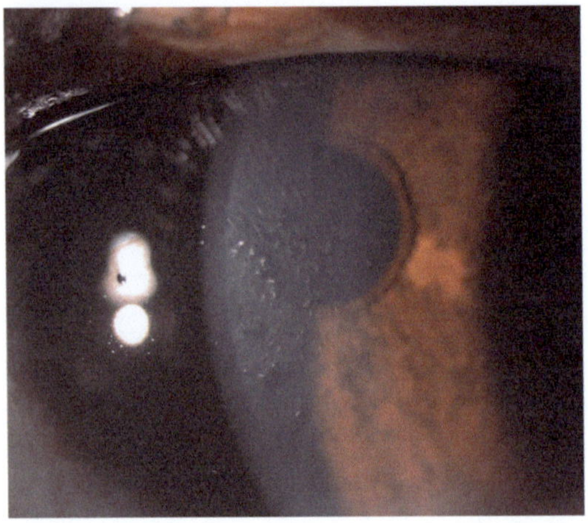

Figure depicting multiple wart-like excrescences in the Descemet's membrane giving a beaten metal appearance characteristic of guttae

References

1. Lemp MA, Zimmerman LE. Conjunctival concretions. Am J Ophthalmol. 1963;55:59–63.
2. Krachmer JH, Mannis MJ, Holland EJ. Cornea. Elsevier Health Sciences; 2013. Chapter 7. p. 78–80.
3. Cavallerano AA. Diagnosis and management of corneal degenerations. Optom Clin. 1992;2(2):57–70.
4. Dougherty PJ, Stark WJ, Gottsch JD. Treatment of Salzmann's nodular degeneration with Nd laser phototherapeutic keratectomy. Am J Ophthalmol. 1996;122(2):263–9.
5. Liu L, Wu J, Geng J, Yuan Z, Huang D. Geographical prevalence and risk factors for pterygium: a systematic review and meta-analysis. BMJ Open. 2013;3:11.
6. Shields JA, Demirci H, Marr BP, Eagle RC Jr, Shields CL. Conjunctival epithelial inclusion cysts: a report of 30 cases and review of the literature. Ophthalmic Plast Reconstr Surg. 2004;20(5):416–20.
7. Fraunfelder FT, Fraunfelder FW. Amiodarone. In: Drug-induced ocular side effects. 7th ed. Philadelphia: Elsevier; 2014. p. 59–68.
8. Latasiewicz MJ, Yushin A, Roth M. Drug-induced corneal deposits: pathogenesis, incidence, and management. Optom Vis Sci. 2015;92(1):89–96.
9. Hope-Ross M, Chell PB, Kervick GN, et al. Amiodarone keratopathy: a study of corneal deposits in 25 patients. Br J Ophthalmol. 1993;77(6):343–6.
10. Cullen AP. Climatic droplet keratopathy. In: Krachmer JH, Mannis MJ, Holland EJ, editors. Cornea. 2nd ed. Philadelphia: Elsevier; 2005. p. 927–35.
11. Lemp MA. Superficial punctate keratitis in dry eye syndromes. Int Ophthalmol Clin. 1973;13(1):213–27.
12. Jeng BH, McLeod SD. Adenoviral keratoconjunctivitis. Curr Opin Ophthalmol. 2003;14(4):420–3.
13. Bron AJ, Williams HP. The desquamation of corneal epithelial cells. Eye (Lond). 1988;2(Pt 3):248–52.
14. Reibaldi M, Longo A, Pulvirenti A, Avitabile T, Reibaldi A. Lipid keratopathy: etiopathogenesis and treatment. Biomed Res Int. 2015;2015:764380.
15. Tananuvat N, Martin T, Loh R, Chirapapaisan C. Conjunctival inclusion cysts after strabismus surgery: incidence and outcomes. J AAPOS. 2011;15(2):165–7.
16. Elhalis H, Azizi B, Jurkunas UV. Fuchs endothelial corneal dystrophy. Ocul Surf. 2010;8(4):173–84.

Corneal Dystrophies

6

Bharat Gurnani, Kirandeep Kaur, Shweta Agarwal,
Bhaskar Srinivasan, and Geetha Iyer

6.1 Introduction

Corneal dystrophies are a group of inherited disorders characterized by bilateral, progressive opacification of the cornea due to the deposition of various materials. These conditions are typically classified based on the layer of the cornea they affect—epithelial, stromal, or endothelial. Corneal dystrophies can significantly impair vision and cause recurrent corneal erosions, leading to pain and discomfort. Understanding the distinct clinical features, genetics, and management strategies for each dystrophy is crucial for effective diagnosis and treatment. This chapter discusses several key corneal dystrophies: lattice corneal dystrophy, granular dystrophy, macular dystrophy, pre-Descemet's dystrophy, Fuchs' corneal dystrophy, congenital hereditary endothelial dystrophy, Reis–Bücklers dystrophy, and posterior polymorphous corneal dystrophy.

6.1.1 Lattice Corneal Dystrophy

Lattice corneal dystrophy (LCD) is characterized by the accumulation of amyloid deposits in the corneal stroma, forming a lattice-like pattern. LCD typically presents in the first or second decade of life with recurrent corneal erosions, decreased visual acuity, and photophobia. Management involves lubricating eye drops for symptom relief, and in severe cases, corneal transplantation may be necessary [1, 2].

B. Gurnani (✉)
Department of Cataract, Cornea, Trauma, External Diseases, Ocular Surface and Refractive Services, Gomabai Netralaya and Research Centre, Neemuch, Madhya Pradesh, India

K. Kaur
Department of Cataract, Pediatric Ophthalmology and Strabismus, Gomabai Netralaya and Research Centre, Neemuch, Madhya Pradesh, India

S. Agarwal · B. Srinivasan · G. Iyer
CJ Shah Cornea Services, Medical Research Foundation, Sankara Nethralaya, Chennai, Tamil Nadu, India

B. Gurnani, K. Kaur (eds.), *Atlas of Cornea*, https://doi.org/10.1007/978-981-96-0013-7_6

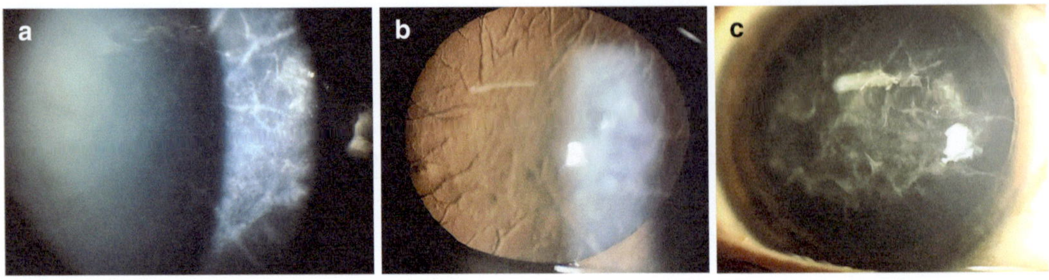

(**a**) Slit, (**b**) retro, and (**c**) diffuse illumination on a slit lamp showing linear radiating thread-like lesions in the anterior to mid-stroma suggestive of lattice corneal dystrophy

6.2 Granular Dystrophy

6.2.1 Diffuse Involvement of Cornea

Granular corneal dystrophy (GCD) is marked by the presence of discrete, breadcrumb-like opacities in the corneal stroma. GCD can be further classified into two types: GCD type 1 (classic) and GCD type 2 (Avellino). These opacities progressively worsen, leading to significant visual impairment. Treatment options include phototherapeutic keratectomy (PTK) and, for advanced cases, corneal transplantation [3, 4].

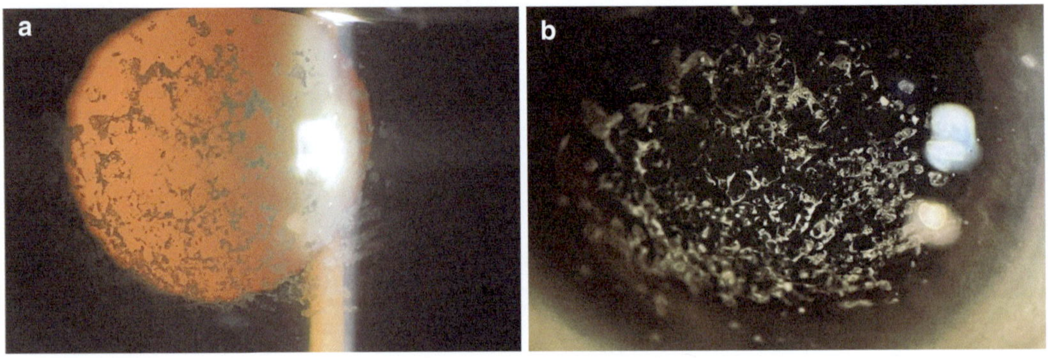

(**a**) Retroillumination and (**b**) diffuse slit lamp picture showing discrete crumb-like opacities in the central anterior stroma with clear intervening spaces suggestive of granular corneal dystrophy

6.2.2 Early Corneal Involvement

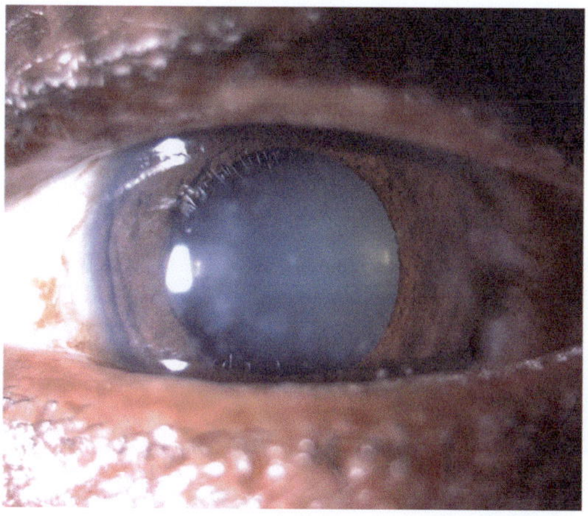

Diffuse slit lamp picture showing discrete crumb-like opacities in the central anterior stroma with clear intervening spaces suggestive of granular corneal dystrophy

6.2.3 Central and Paracentral Corneal Involvement

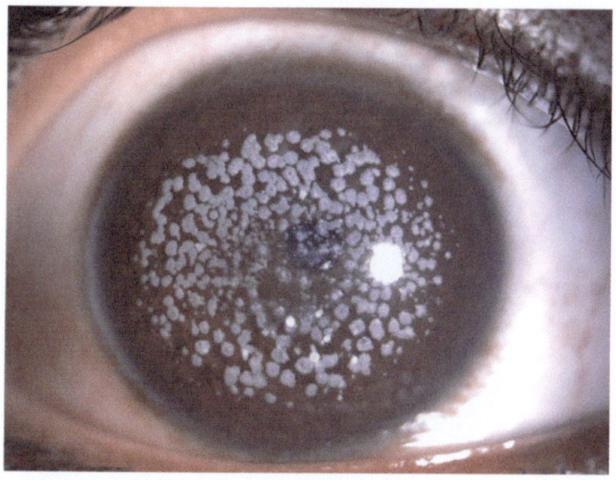

Diffuse slit lamp picture showing discrete crumb-like opacities in the central anterior stroma with clear intervening spaces suggestive of granular corneal dystrophy

6.2.4 Granular Dystrophy with Mature Cataract

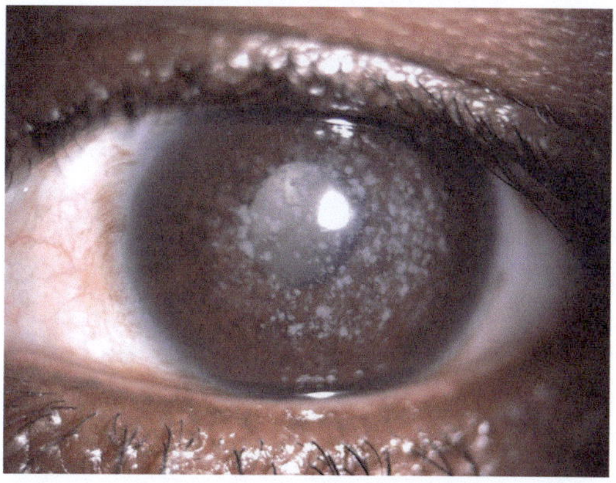

Diffuse slit lamp picture showing discrete crumb-like opacities in the central anterior stroma with clear intervening spaces suggestive of granular corneal dystrophy

6.2.5 Focal Central Corneal Involvement

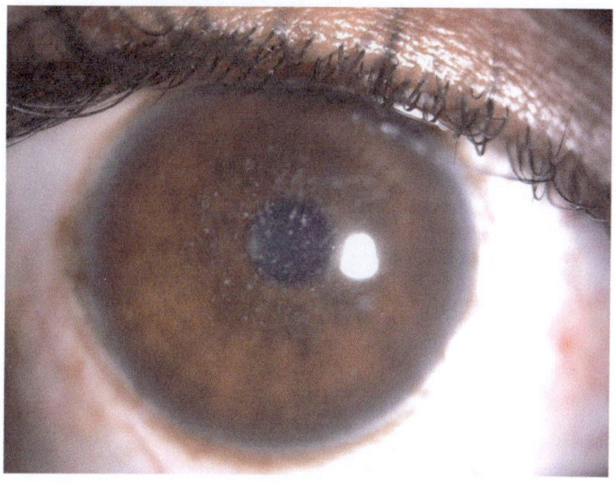

Diffuse slit lamp picture showing discrete crumb-like opacities in the central anterior stroma with clear intervening spaces suggestive of granular corneal dystrophy

6.3 Macular Dystrophy

6.3.1 Stromal Haze with Mature Cataract

Macular corneal dystrophy (MCD) is an autosomal recessive disorder characterized by diffuse stromal haze and focal macular opacities. MCD often presents in the first decade of life and progressively worsens, causing significant visual impairment. Given the diffuse nature of the opacities, corneal transplantation is often required to restore vision [5].

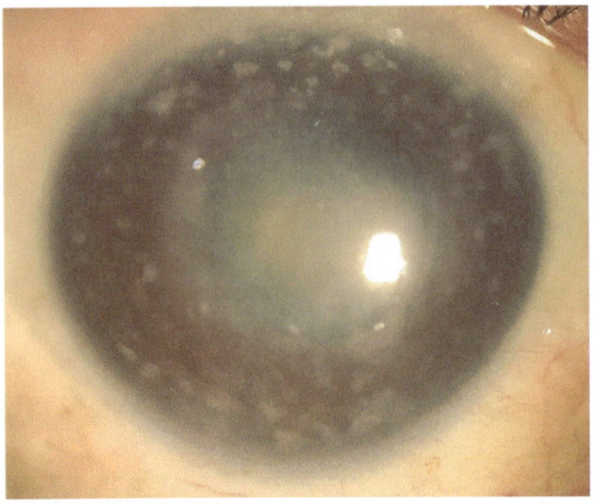

Diffuse slit lamp picture showing stromal opacities with indistinct borders and intervening haze extending up to the limbus

6.3.2 Central Macular Dystrophy

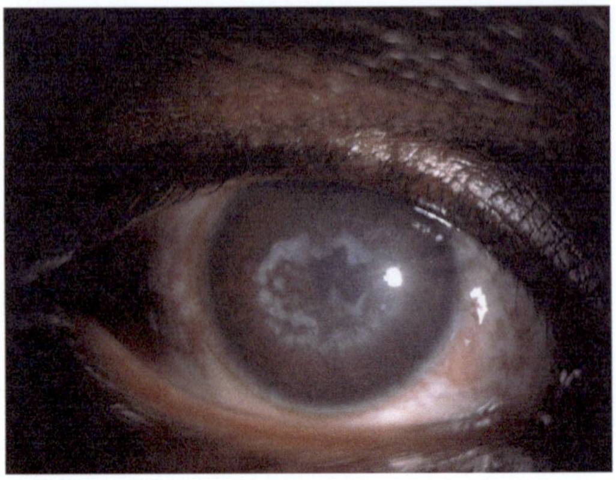

Diffuse slit lamp picture showing stromal opacities with indistinct borders and intervening haze extending up to the limbus

6.3.3 Pre- and Post-Phototherapeutic Keratectomy

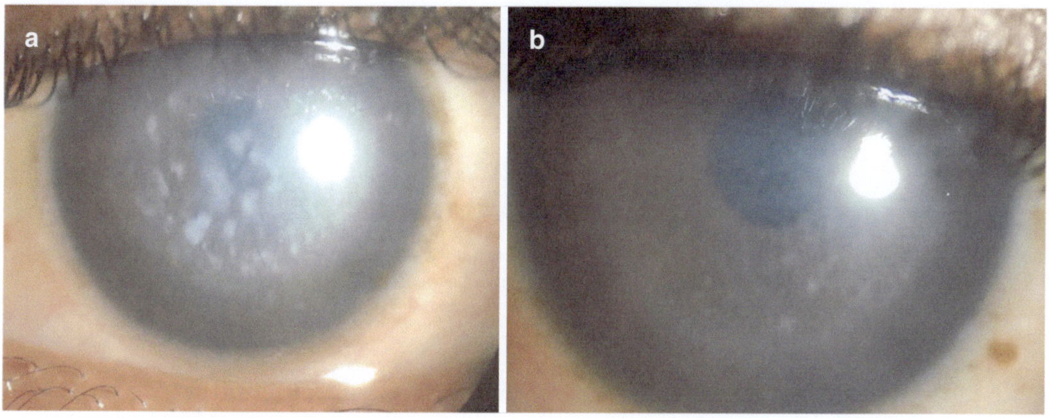

(**a**) Diffuse slit lamp picture showing stromal opacities with indistinct borders and intervening haze. (**b**) Relatively clear cornea with no opacities seen following phototherapeutic keratectomy in macular corneal dystrophy

6.3.4 Pre-Descemet's Dystrophy

Pre-Descemet's dystrophy is a rare corneal condition characterized by fine, superficial, grayish opacities just anterior to Descemet's membrane. These opacities are typically asymptomatic and do not significantly impact vision. Regular monitoring is usually sufficient, and intervention is rarely necessary unless complications arise [6].

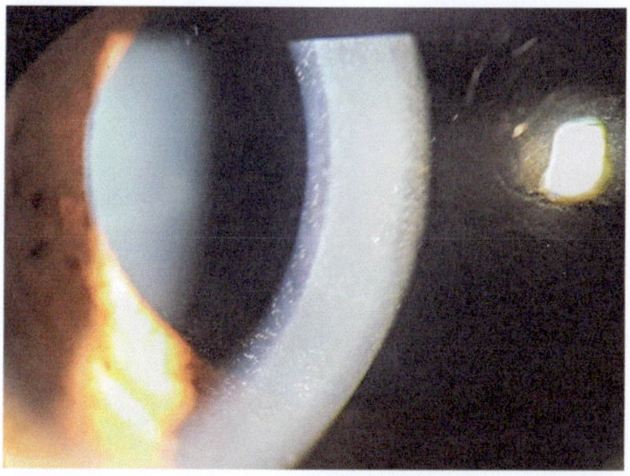

Slit lamp picture showing multiple small discrete opacities in the stroma just anterior to the Descemet's membrane

6.3.5 Fuchs' Corneal Dystrophy

Fuchs' corneal dystrophy (FCD) is a progressive disorder affecting the corneal endothelium, leading to endothelial cell loss and subsequent corneal edema. Symptoms typically present in the fourth or fifth decade of life and include blurred vision, glare, and halos around lights. Management strategies for FCD include hypertonic saline drops for mild cases and endothelial keratoplasty or penetrating keratoplasty for advanced cases [7, 8].

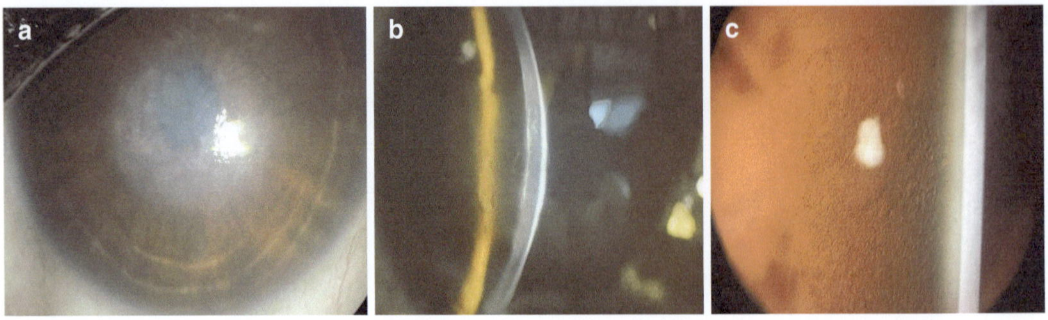

(**a**) Diffuse slit lamp picture showing central haze and edema. (**b**) Slit lamp picture showing minimally increased corneal thickness in the central cornea as compared to the periphery. (**c**) Retroillumination showing classical "beaten metal appearance" in FECD

6.3.6 Congenital Hereditary Endothelial Dystrophy

Congenital hereditary endothelial dystrophy (CHED) is a rare, autosomal recessive condition presenting at birth or early childhood with diffuse corneal clouding and edema due to endothelial dysfunction. CHED often requires early surgical intervention, such as endothelial keratoplasty or penetrating keratoplasty, to restore vision [9].

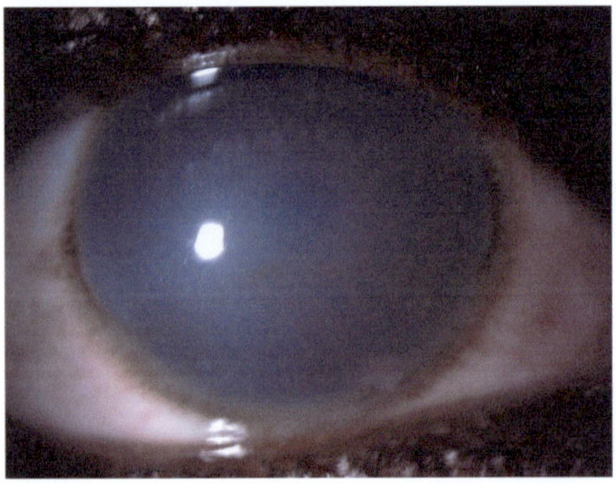

Diffuse illumination slit lamp image of a patient depicting severe corneal opacification with thickening of the Descemet membrane

6.4 Reis–Bucklers Dystrophy

6.4.1 Geographic Subepithelial Opacities: Dense Centrally

Reis–Bücklers dystrophy is an autosomal dominant condition characterized by the deposition of fibrous material beneath the corneal epithelium, leading to recurrent corneal erosions and decreased visual acuity. Management includes lubricating eye drops and therapeutic contact lenses for symptom relief, with PTK or corneal transplantation for severe cases [10].

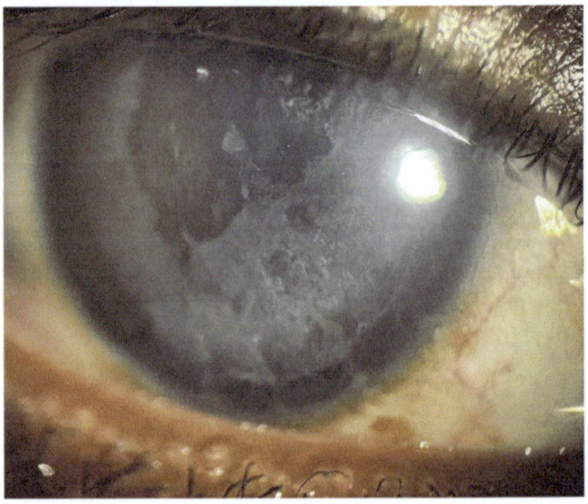

Slit lamp picture showing diffuse sub-epithelial haze with gray–white geographic subepithelial opacities, most dense centrally

6.4.2 Total Corneal Involvement

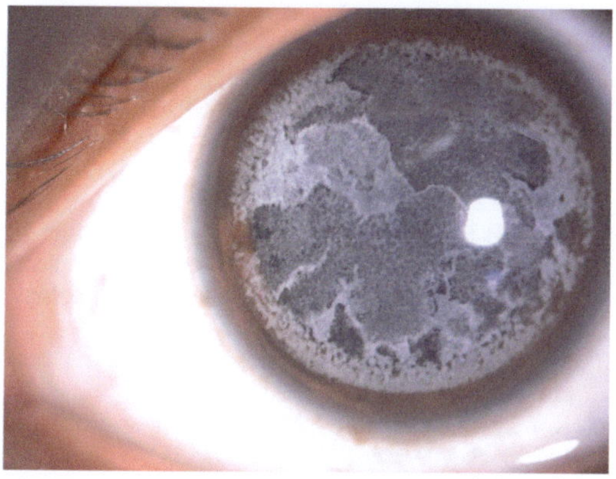

Slit lamp picture showing diffuse sub-epithelial haze with gray–white geographic subepithelial opacities, most dense centrally and forming a reticular pattern

6.4.3 Superficial Corneal Involvement

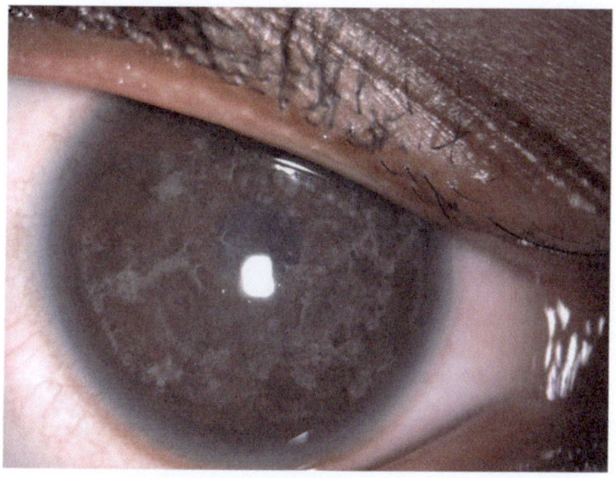

Slit lamp picture showing diffuse sub-epithelial haze with gray–white geographic subepithelial opacities

6.5 Posterior Polymorphous Corneal Dystrophy

6.5.1 Endothelial Vesicular Lesions

Posterior polymorphous corneal dystrophy (PPCD) is a rare, autosomal dominant disorder affecting the corneal endothelium and Descemet's membrane. PPCD can present with variable clinical features, including corneal edema and peripheral anterior synechiae. Management focuses on controlling intraocular pressure and addressing corneal edema, with endothelial keratoplasty considered for severe cases [11].

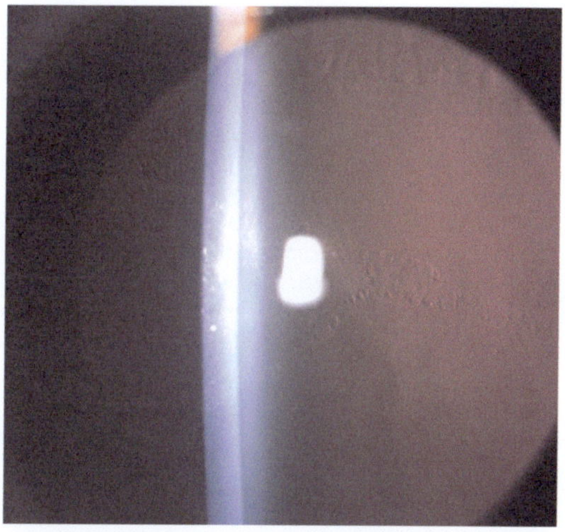

Slit lamp image in retroillumination depicting endothelial vesicular lesions and band lesions suggestive of posterior polymorphous corneal dystrophy

6.6 Posterior Polymorphous Corneal Dystrophy

6.6.1 Band-Shaped Lesion

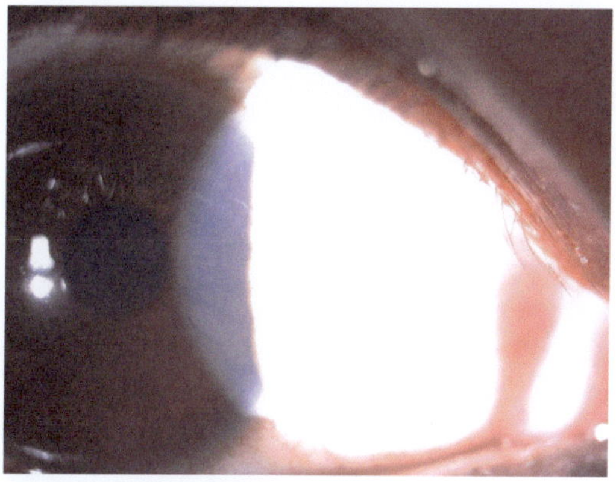

Diffuse slit lamp illumination image depicting subtle vesicular, band-like endothelial lesions

References

1. Weiss JS, Møller HU, Aldave AJ, Seitz B, Bredrup C, Kivela T, et al. IC3D classification of corneal dystrophies—edition 2. Cornea. 2015;34(2):117–59.
2. Krachmer JH, Mannis MJ, Holland EJ. Cornea. Elsevier Health Sciences; 2013. Chapter 7. p. 78–80.
3. Lisch W, Steuhl KP, Schlotzer-Schrehardt U, et al. Macular corneal dystrophy: mutational spectrum and deposition pattern of keratan sulfate proteoglycan. Invest Ophthalmol Vis Sci. 2013;54(6):3909–19.
4. Aldave AJ, Sonmez B. Elucidating the molecular genetic basis of the corneal dystrophies: are we there yet? Arch Ophthalmol. 2007;125(1):101–15.
5. Weiss JS, Møller HU, Lisch W, Kinoshita S, Aldave AJ, Belin MW, et al. The IC3D classification of the corneal dystrophies. Cornea. 2008;27(Suppl):2.
6. Aldave AJ, Yellore VS. Corneal endothelial dystrophies: clinical, pathological, and genetic aspects. Am J Ophthalmol. 2014;158(2):226–37.
7. Gottsch JD, Sundin OH, Liu SH, Jun AS, Broman KW, Stark WJ, et al. Inheritance of a novel COL8A2 mutation defines a distinct early-onset subtype of Fuchs corneal dystrophy. Invest Ophthalmol Vis Sci. 2005;46(6):1934–9.
8. Liskova P, Prescott Q, Bhattacharya SS, Tuft SJ. British family with early-onset Fuchs endothelial corneal dystrophy associated with p.Leu450Trp COL8A2. Eye (Lond). 2007;21(7):865–70.
9. Nair SP, Elhaik E, Edlund CK, Schmedt T, Miller K, Tribbick D, et al. Molecular genetic study of congenital hereditary endothelial dystrophy. Ophthalmology. 2014;121(12):2339–44.
10. Meek KM, Knupp C. Corneal structure and transparency. Prog Retin Eye Res. 2015;49:1–16.
11. Krafchak CM, Pawar H, Moroi SE, Sugar A, Lichter PR, Mackey DA, et al. Mutations in TCF8 cause posterior polymorphous corneal dystrophy and ectopic expression of COL4A3 by corneal endothelial cells. Am J Hum Genet. 2005;77(2):241–51.

7 Corneal Ectatic Diseases

Bharat Gurnani, Kirandeep Kaur, and Anitha Venugopal

7.1 Introduction

Corneal ectatic diseases encompass a group of progressive, noninflammatory disorders characterized by the thinning and bulging of the cornea. These conditions can lead to significant visual impairment due to the irregular shape of the cornea, which distorts vision. This chapter explores several key corneal ectatic diseases: keratoconus, pellucid marginal degeneration, keratoglobus, Terrien's marginal degeneration, as well as management strategies such as corneal collagen cross-linking with riboflavin, treatment for corneal hydrops, and the use of scleral contact lenses in keratoconus.

B. Gurnani
Department of Cataract, Cornea, Trauma, External Diseases, Ocular Surface and Refractive Services, Gomabai Netralaya and Research Centre, Neemuch, Madhya Pradesh, India

K. Kaur (✉)
Department of Cataract, Pediatric Ophthalmology and Strabismus, Gomabai Netralaya and Research Centre, Neemuch, Madhya Pradesh, India

A. Venugopal
Cornea, Ocular Surface, Trauma and Refractive, Services, Aravind Eye Hospital and Postgraduate Institute of Ophthalmology, Tirunelveli, Tamil Nadu, India

7.2 Keratoconus

7.2.1 Vogt's Striae

Keratoconus is the most common corneal ectatic disorder, characterized by progressive thinning and conical protrusion of the cornea. It typically presents in adolescence or early adulthood with symptoms such as blurred vision, glare, and light sensitivity. The condition can lead to significant astigmatism and myopia. Management includes rigid gas-permeable contact lenses, scleral lenses, and, in severe cases, corneal transplantation. Corneal collagen cross-linking (CXL) has emerged as a key treatment to halt the progression of keratoconus by strengthening corneal collagen fibers [1, 2].

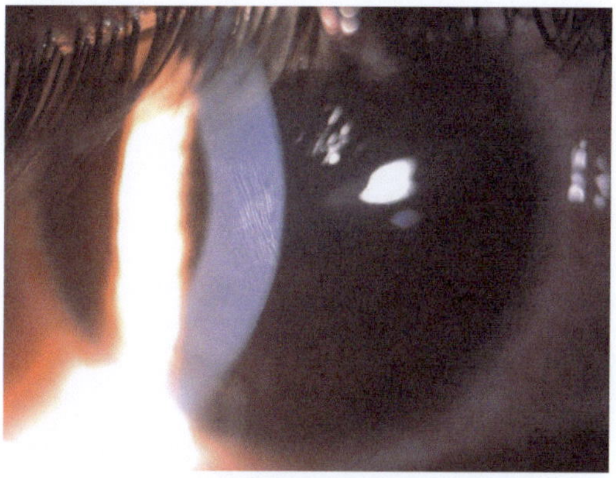

Slit lamp image of a patient depicting vertical lines in the posterior stroma and Descemet's membrane of cornea suggestive of Vogt's striae seen in keratoconus

B. Gurnani, K. Kaur (eds.), *Atlas of Cornea*, https://doi.org/10.1007/978-981-96-0013-7_7

7.2.2 Conical Corneal Protrusion

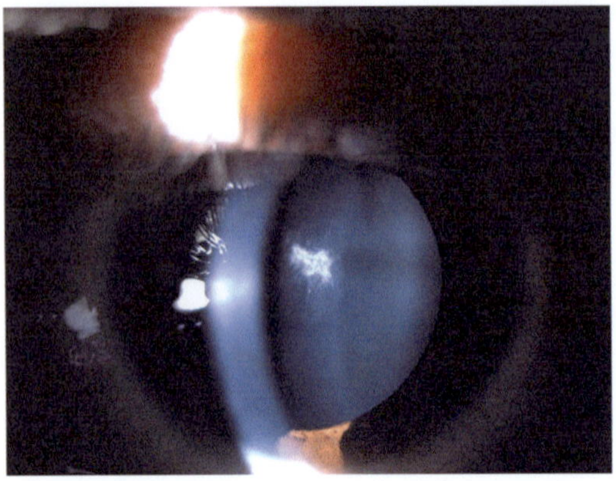

Diffuse illumination slit lamp image of a patient depicting conical protrusion of the cornea along with anterior subcapsular cataract in a patient with keratoconus

7.2.3 Post-Collagen Cross-Linking with Riboflavin: Infectious Keratitis

Corneal collagen cross-linking (CXL) with riboflavin is a treatment that has revolutionized the management of corneal ectatic diseases, particularly keratoconus. CXL involves the application of riboflavin (vitamin B2) to the cornea, followed by ultraviolet-A (UV-A) light exposure. This process increases the biomechanical strength of the cornea by creating additional covalent bonds between collagen fibers, thus halting the progression of ectasia. CXL is effective in stabilizing the cornea and reducing the need for corneal transplantation [3, 4].

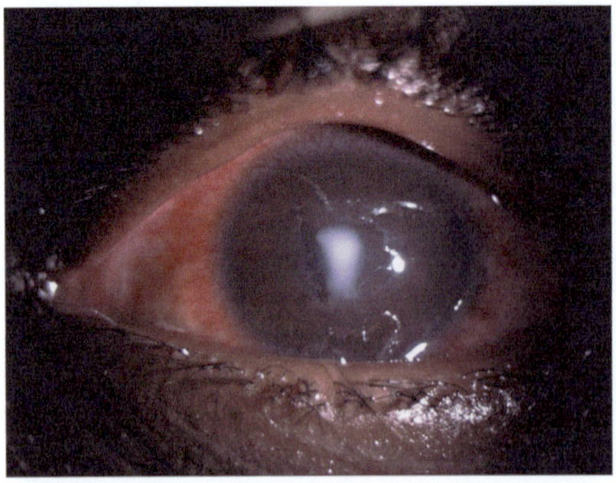

Diffuse illumination slit lamp image of a patient depicting a central epithelial defect with anterior stromal infiltrate in a patient with keratoconus post-corneal collagen cross-linking

7.2.4 Corneal Scar Post-Hydrops

Corneal hydrops is a complication of advanced ectatic diseases, where there is a sudden break in Descemet's membrane, leading to an influx of aqueous humor into the corneal stroma. This results in acute corneal edema, pain, and severe vision loss. Management includes hypertonic saline drops, bandage contact lenses, and anti-inflammatory medications to reduce corneal edema. Surgical options may be considered in refractory cases [5].

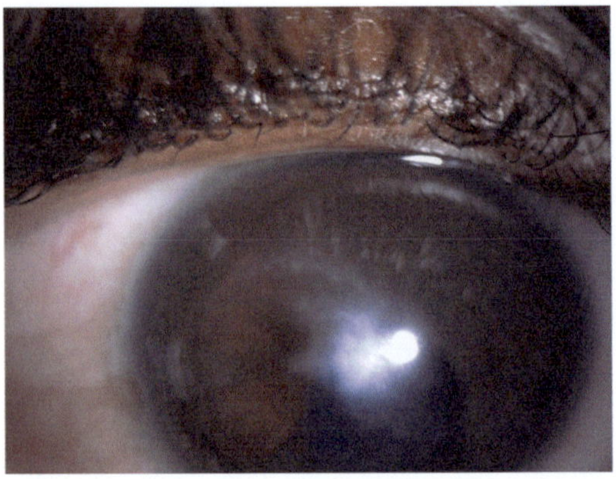

Diffuse illumination slit lamp image of a patient depicting central macular corneal scar in a keratoconus patient with old corneal hydrops

7.2.5 Scleral Contact Lens in Keratoconus

Scleral contact lenses have become a mainstay in the management of keratoconus, particularly in patients with advanced disease where traditional contact lenses are inadequate. These large-diameter lenses vault over the cornea and rest on the sclera, providing a smooth optical surface that improves vision. Scleral lenses are particularly beneficial for patients with irregular corneal surfaces, as they provide comfort and stability while correcting refractive errors [6].

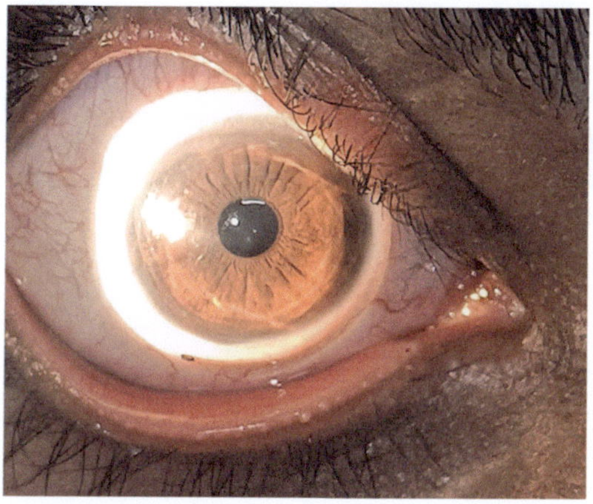

Digital image depicting rehabilitation of a keratoconus patient with contact lenses

7.2.6 Post-Deep Anterior Lamellar Keratoplasty

Deep anterior lamellar keratoplasty (DALK) is a surgical procedure used to treat keratoconus by replacing the diseased corneal stroma while preserving the patient's own endothelium. This technique reduces the risk of endothelial rejection and can lead to excellent visual outcomes and graft survival [7].

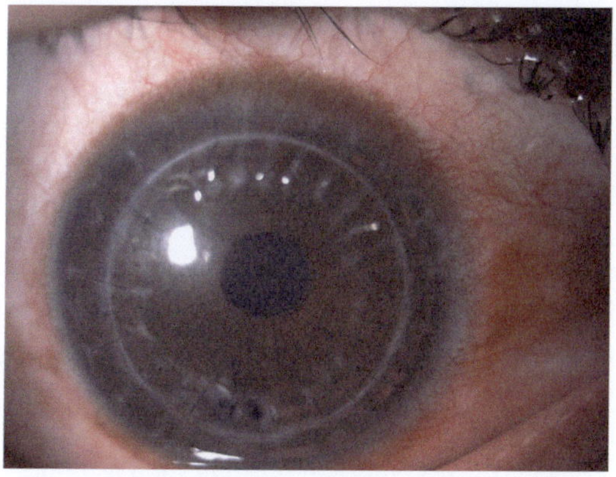

Diffuse illumination slit lamp image of a patient depicting well-opposed DALK graft in a patient with advanced keratoconus

7.2.7 Post-Optical Penetrating Keratoplasty

Post-optical penetrating keratoplasty (PK) in keratoconus involves replacing the conical central part of the cornea with a donor graft to restore visual acuity. This procedure is often indicated for advanced keratoconus when other treatments fail, leading to significant improvement in vision and quality of life [8].

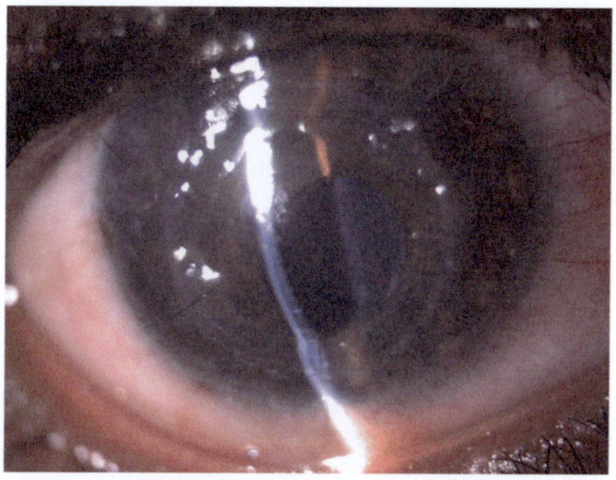

Diffuse illumination slit lamp image of the advanced keratoconus patient post-optical keratoplasty depicting 7.5 mm clear graft, well-opposed graft host junction with intact sutures

7.2.8 Keratoglobus

Keratoglobus is a rare ectatic disorder characterized by diffuse thinning and globular protrusion of the cornea, affecting the entire cornea. Patients with keratoglobus are prone to corneal rupture even with minor trauma due to the extreme thinning. Management focuses on protecting the cornea with rigid or scleral contact lenses and, in severe cases, lamellar or penetrating keratoplasty [9].

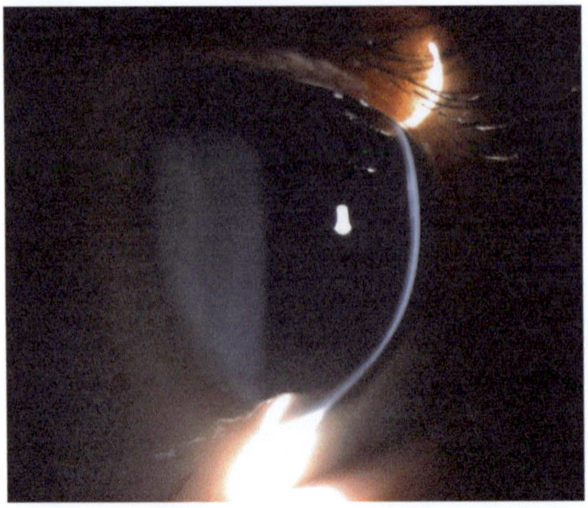

Diffuse illumination image of a patient depicting globally thin and ectatic cornea, clinically suggestive of keratoglobus

7.2.9 Pellucid Marginal Degeneration

Pellucid marginal degeneration (PMD) is characterized by inferior peripheral corneal thinning, leading to a band of thinning typically 1–2 mm wide, located 1–2 mm above the inferior limbus. This condition results in high against-the-rule astigmatism and irregular corneal topography. Unlike keratoconus, the central cornea remains relatively clear. Treatment includes specialty contact lenses such as scleral lenses and surgical options like crescentic lamellar keratoplasty and CXL [10, 11].

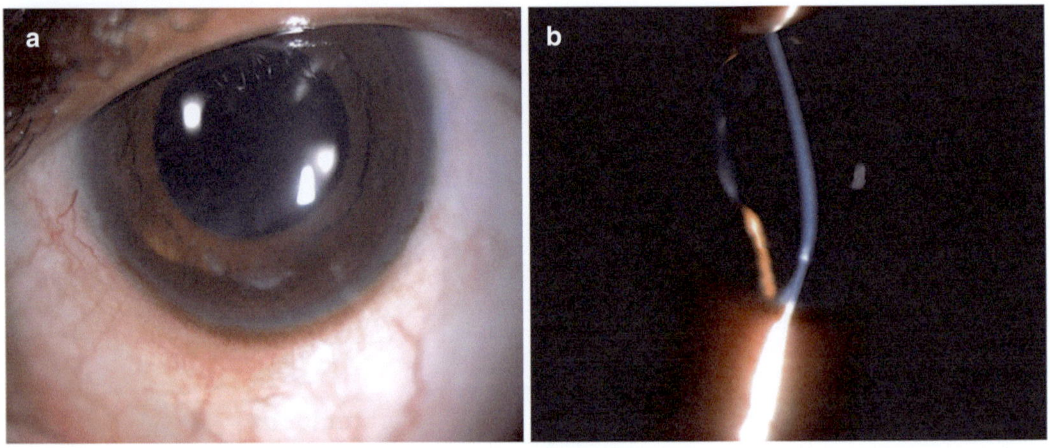

(**a**) Diffuse illumination slit lamp image of a patient depicting inferior band of corneal thinning; (**b**) slit lamp image of the same patient depicting bending of rays in the inferior cornea, suggestive of pellucid marginal degeneration

7.2.10 Terrien's Marginal Degeneration

Terrien's marginal degeneration is a rare, slowly progressive ectatic condition that typically affects older adults. It involves peripheral corneal thinning with a clear zone separating the thinning from the limbus and a vascularized pannus overlying the thinned area. Patients may present with visual impairment due to irregular astigmatism. Management includes the use of specialty contact lenses and, in advanced cases, surgical options such as lamellar keratoplasty [12].

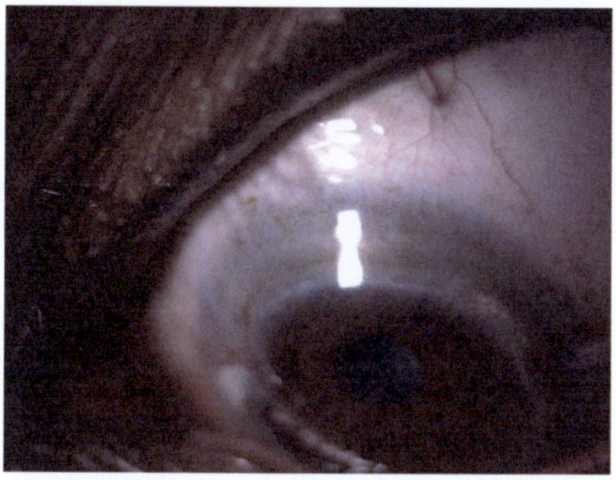

Diffuse illumination slit lamp image of a patient depicting superior corneal thinning and lipid deposits in a case with Terrien's marginal degeneration

References

1. Rabinowitz YS. Keratoconus. Surv Ophthalmol. 1998;42(4):297–319.
2. Wittig-Silva C, Chan E, Hicks N, et al. A randomized controlled trial of corneal collagen cross-linking in progressive keratoconus: three-year results. Ophthalmology. 2014;121(4):812–21.
3. Wollensak G, Spoerl E, Seiler T. Riboflavin/ultraviolet-A-induced collagen crosslinking for the treatment of keratoconus. Am J Ophthalmol. 2003;135(5):620–7.
4. Hersh PS, Greenstein SA, Fry KL. Corneal collagen crosslinking for keratoconus and corneal ectasia: one-year results. J Cataract Refract Surg. 2011;37(1):149–60.
5. Macsai MS, Shiloach M. Use of intracameral gas injection to treat acute corneal hydrops. Cornea. 2000;19(2):272–3.
6. Barnett M, Mannis MJ. Contact lenses in the management of keratoconus. Cornea. 2011;30(12):1510–6.
7. Anwar M, Teichmann KD. Big-bubble technique to bare Descemet's membrane in anterior lamellar keratoplasty. J Cataract Refract Surg. 2002;28(3):398–403.
8. Price FW Jr, Price MO. Long-term outcomes of penetrating keratoplasty for keratoconus. Trans Am Ophthalmol Soc. 2005;103:189–203.
9. Sherwin T, Brookes NH. Morphological changes in keratoconus: pathology or pathogenesis. Clin Experiment Ophthalmol. 2004;32(6):211–7.
10. Krachmer JH, Feder RS, Belin MW. Pellucid marginal corneal degeneration. Ophthalmology. 1984;91(1):26–31.
11. Mohammadpour M, Masoumi A, Mirghorbani M, et al. Updates on managements for keratoconus. J Curr Ophthalmol. 2018;30(2):110–24.
12. Krachmer JH, Mannis MJ, Holland EJ. Cornea. Elsevier Health Sciences; 2013. Chapter 47. p. 591–7.

Systemic Disorders with Corneal Involvement

8

Kirandeep Kaur and Bharat Gurnani

8.1 Introduction

Systemic disorders often present with multifaceted clinical manifestations, including ocular involvement. The cornea, being a transparent and avascular structure, can be affected in various systemic conditions, leading to significant visual impairment. Understanding the corneal manifestations of these systemic disorders is crucial for early diagnosis, appropriate management, and improving patient outcomes. This section delves into various systemic disorders with corneal involvement, highlighting congenital hereditary stromal dystrophy in lysosomal storage disorders, epibulbar dermoid in Goldenhar syndrome, congenital sclerocornea secondary to rubella, exposure keratopathy in Hansen's disease, corneal perforation secondary to peripheral ulcerative keratitis in Wegener's granulomatosis, nutritional keratopathy secondary to protein energy malnutrition, adherent leukoma in Peter's anomaly, and acute hydrops in Down syndrome.

K. Kaur
Department of Cataract, Pediatric Ophthalmology and Strabismus, Gomabai Netralaya and Research Centre, Neemuch, Madhya Pradesh, India

B. Gurnani (✉)
Department of Cataract, Cornea, Trauma, External Diseases, Ocular Surface and Refractive Services, Gomabai Netralaya and Research Centre, Neemuch, Madhya Pradesh, India

8.2 Congenital Hereditary Stromal Dystrophy in Lysosomal Storage Disorder

Congenital hereditary stromal dystrophy (CHSD) is a rare, nonprogressive corneal dystrophy characterized by diffuse cloudiness of the stroma, resulting in visual impairment from birth. In the context of lysosomal storage disorders, CHSD can be associated with systemic metabolic abnormalities where defective lysosomal enzymes lead to the accumulation of substrates within the corneal stroma, exacerbating cloudiness and visual disturbances. These conditions, such as mucopolysaccharidoses and other storage diseases, highlight the systemic nature of the disorder and the necessity for a multidisciplinary treatment approach, often involving enzyme replacement therapy and corneal transplantation [1].

B. Gurnani, K. Kaur (eds.), *Atlas of Cornea*, https://doi.org/10.1007/978-981-96-0013-7_8

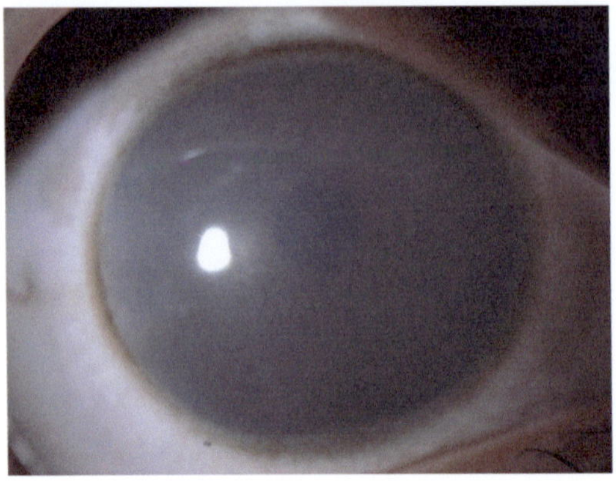

Diffuse illumination slit lamp image of a patient depicting stromal edema with haze in a patient with congenital hereditary stromal dystrophy

8.3 Epibulbar Dermoid Goldenhar Syndrome

Goldenhar syndrome, or oculoauriculovertebral spectrum, is a congenital condition characterized by craniofacial anomalies, including epibulbar dermoids. These benign growths are typically located at the corneoscleral limbus and can cause astigmatism and visual axis obstruction. The dermoids can vary in size and may be associated with other ocular abnormalities such as microphthalmia and coloboma. Surgical removal is often necessary to improve cosmesis and visual function, and ongoing ophthalmic evaluations are crucial for managing associated refractive errors and amblyopia [2].

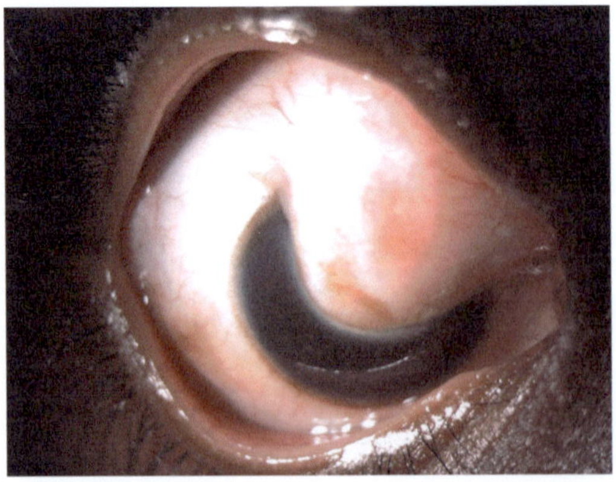

Diffuse illumination slit lamp image of a patient depicting congenital epibulbar dermoid in a child with Goldenhar syndrome

8.4 Congenital Sclerocornea Secondary to Rubella

Congenital sclerocornea, characterized by the opacity of the peripheral or entire cornea, can result from intrauterine infections such as rubella. The rubella virus can disrupt normal ocular development, leading to sclerocornea and other ocular abnormalities like cataracts, microphthalmia, and glaucoma. Management focuses on addressing the visual impairment through surgical interventions, including corneal transplantation, and treating associated ocular conditions to improve visual outcomes [3].

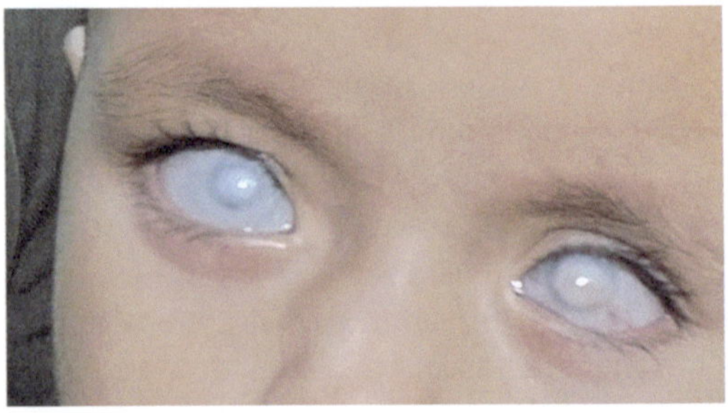

Digital gross image of a patient depicting congenital sclerocornea secondary to maternal rubella infection

8.5 Exposure Keratopathy in Hansen's Disease

Hansen's disease (leprosy) can lead to exposure keratopathy due to facial nerve involvement, causing lagophthalmos and reduced blink reflex. The resultant exposure of the cornea leads to dryness, ulceration, and potential secondary infections. Management includes lubricating eye drops, protective measures such as tarsorrhaphy, and addressing underlying leprosy with multidrug therapy to prevent further nerve damage and progression of the disease [4].

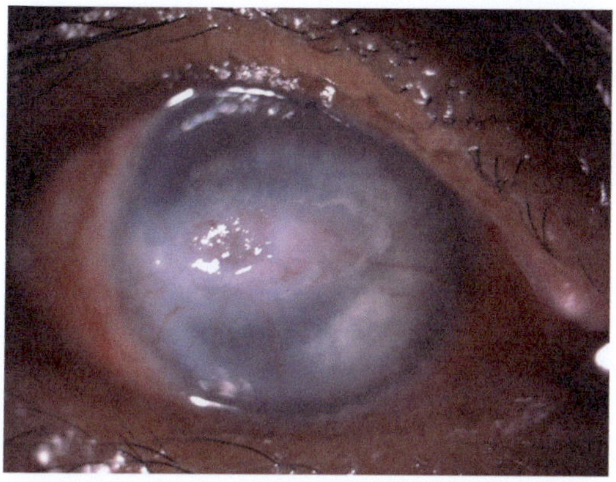

Digital gross image of a patient with Hansen's disease depicting central exposure keratopathy with thinning and superficial vascularization

8.6 Corneal Perforation Secondary to Peripheral Ulcerative Keratitis in a Patient with Wegner's Granulomatosis

Wegener's granulomatosis, an autoimmune vasculitis now known as granulomatosis with polyangiitis, can cause peripheral ulcerative keratitis (PUK), leading to corneal perforation. The inflammatory process involves the peripheral cornea, resulting in thinning and ulceration. Immediate management involves systemic immunosuppression to control the underlying vasculitis and surgical intervention, such as corneal gluing or keratoplasty, to restore corneal integrity and prevent vision loss [5].

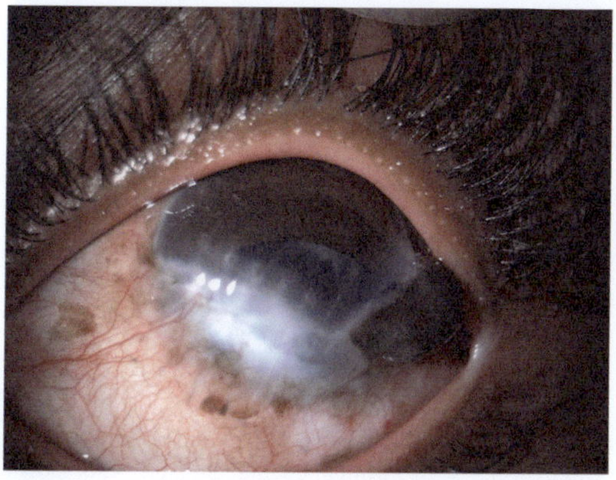

Digital gross image of a patient depicting corneal perforation in a long-standing peripheral ulcerative keratitis secondary to Wegner's granulomatosis

8.7 Nutritional Keratopathy Secondary to Protein Energy Malnutrition

Protein energy malnutrition (PEM) can lead to nutritional keratopathy, characterized by corneal xerosis, ulceration, and potential perforation due to deficiencies in essential nutrients like vitamin A. This condition is prevalent in developing countries where malnutrition is common. Management includes nutritional rehabilitation with vitamin supplementation, especially vitamin A, and addressing any secondary infections or complications to restore corneal health and prevent blindness [6].

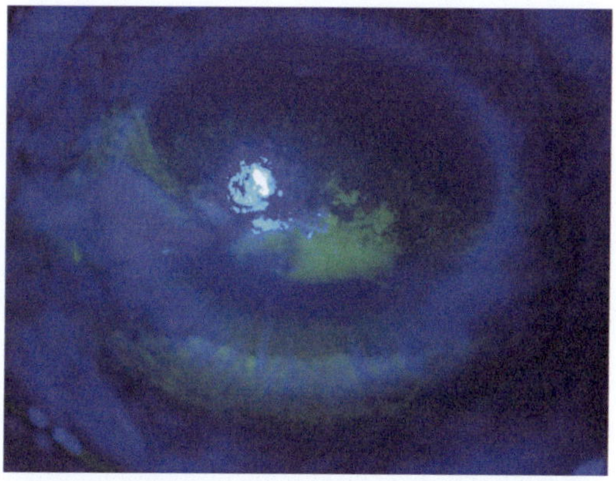

Digital cobalt blue image of a patient depicting central keratopathy with inferior pannus secondary to protein energy malnutrition

8.8 Aqueous Deficiency Dry Eye in a Case of Rheumatoid Arthritis

Aqueous deficiency dry eye in rheumatoid arthritis results from inflammation-induced damage to the lacrimal glands, leading to reduced tear production. This condition causes severe dryness, irritation, and potential corneal damage, necessitating treatments like artificial tears, anti-inflammatory medications, and punctal plugs to improve tear retention and ocular comfort [7].

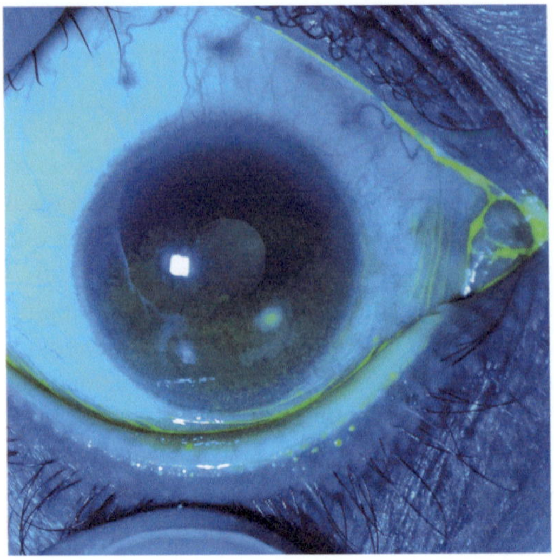

Digital illumination gross cobalt blue filter slit lamp image of a patient with rheumatoid arthritis under fluorescein staining depicting diffuse punctate corneal erosions, mild conjunctival staining, and caruncular staining suggestive of aqueous deficiency dry eyes

8.9 Adherent Leucoma in Peter's Anomaly

Peter's anomaly is a congenital corneal opacity characterized by central corneal leukoma, often with adhesions between the cornea and the iris or lens. This condition can result in significant visual impairment from birth. Management involves surgical interventions such as penetrating keratoplasty to clear the visual axis and ongoing ophthalmic care to address associated anomalies like glaucoma and cataracts, improving visual prognosis [7].

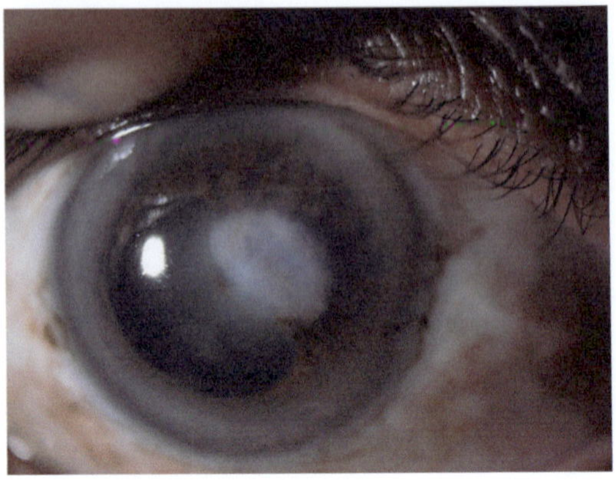

Digital image of a patient depicting congenital adherent leukoma in a case of Peter's anomaly

8.10 Acute Hydrops in Down Syndrome

Acute corneal hydrops, characterized by sudden corneal edema due to a break in Descemet's membrane, can occur in individuals with Down syndrome. The predisposition to keratoconus in Down syndrome increases the risk of acute hydrops. Management involves supportive measures such as hypertonic saline drops, bandage contact lenses, and in severe cases, surgical interventions like intracorneal ring segments or keratoplasty to restore corneal integrity and visual function [8, 9].

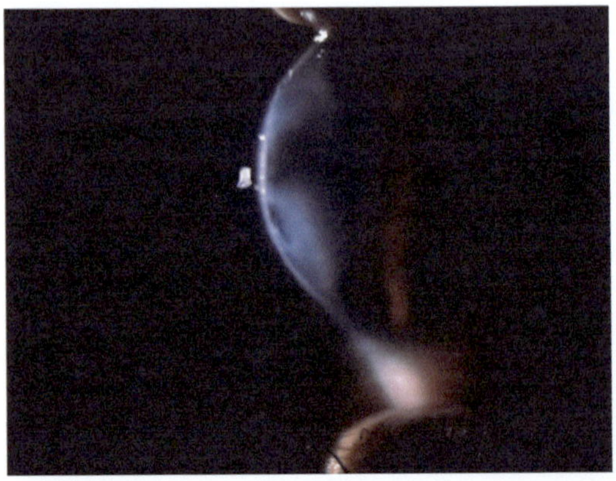

Digital side on the image of a patient depicting acute corneal hydrops with stromal edema affected with Down syndrome

References

1. Kim JE, Kim SM. Advances in the understanding and treatment of congenital hereditary stromal dystrophy. Ophthalmology. 2022;129(2):195–203.
2. Lee H, Lee SH. Clinical management of epibulbar dermoids in Goldenhar syndrome. J Pediatr Ophthalmol Strabismus. 2021;58(5):317–24.
3. Smith AG, Smith GL. Ocular complications of congenital rubella syndrome. Am J Ophthalmol. 2023;235:45–54.
4. Brown RP, Brown DL. Exposure keratopathy in Hansen's disease: a review. Cornea. 2021;40(8):1050–8.
5. Gupta M, Gupta SK. Peripheral ulcerative keratitis in Wegener's granulomatosis. Br J Ophthalmol. 2022;106(3):385–90.
6. Patel V, Patel RM. Nutritional keratopathy: the impact of protein energy malnutrition. J Clin Nutr Metab. 2023;12(2):102–10.
7. Lemp MA, Foulks GN. The definition and classification of dry eye disease: report of the Definition and Classification Subcommittee of the International Dry Eye WorkShop. Ocul Surf. 2007;5(2):75–92.
8. Thomas JE, Thomas DS. Peter's anomaly: current perspectives on diagnosis and management. Clin Ophthalmol. 2021;15:345–53.
9. Johnson LM, Johnson PH. Acute corneal hydrops in Down syndrome patients with keratoconus. Int J Ophthalmol. 2022;14(4):652–8.

Viral Infectious Diseases of the Cornea

9

Radhika Natarajan, Madhuvanthi Mohan, Bharat Gurnani, and Kirandeep Kaur

9.1 Introduction

Viral infectious diseases of the cornea encompass a range of conditions caused by various viruses, each presenting unique clinical features and requiring specific management approaches. These infections can lead to significant morbidity, impacting vision and quality of life. This introduction will highlight key conditions: HSV blepharokeratoconjunctivitis, herpetic viral keratitis, dendritic HSV keratitis, adenoviral subepithelial keratitis, viral stromal keratitis, viral keratouveitis, active herpes zoster nummular keratitis, recurrent herpes simplex keratitis, and viral keratitis with secondary bacterial infiltrate.

R. Natarajan (✉) · M. Mohan
Department of Cornea and Refractive Surgery, Sankara Netralaya Medical Research Foundation, Chennai, Tamil Nadu, India
e-mail: drnr@snmail.org

B. Gurnani
Department of Cataract, Cornea, Trauma, External Diseases, Ocular Surface and Refractive Services, Gomabai Netralaya and Research Centre, Neemuch, Madhya Pradesh, India

K. Kaur
Department of Cataract, Pediatric Ophthalmology and Strabismus, Gomabai Netralaya and Research Centre, Neemuch, Madhya Pradesh, India

9.2 Herpes Simplex Virus Manifestations

9.2.1 Blepharokeratoconjunctivitis

Herpes simplex virus (HSV) blepharokeratoconjunctivitis is an infection involving the eyelids, conjunctiva, and cornea. It typically presents with vesicular lesions on the eyelids, conjunctival injection, and epithelial keratitis. Diagnosis is often clinical, supported by viral cultures or polymerase chain reaction (PCR) testing. Management includes antiviral agents like acyclovir to reduce viral replication and mitigate symptoms [1, 2].

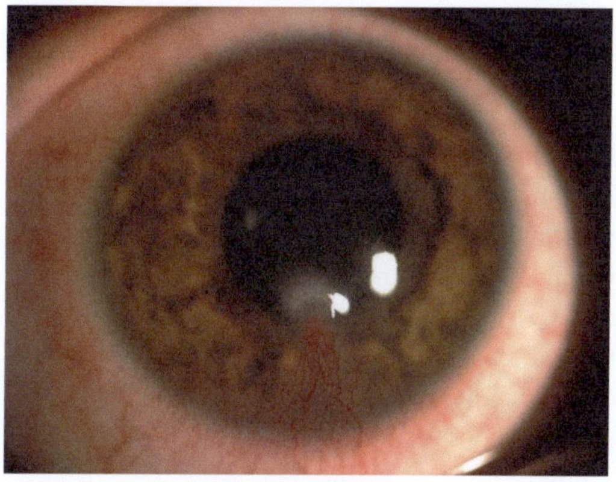

Diffuse illumination slit lamp image of a patient depicting 2 × 2 mm corneal infiltrate paracentrally at 6 o'clock position with superficial vascularization

B. Gurnani, K. Kaur (eds.), *Atlas of Cornea*, https://doi.org/10.1007/978-981-96-0013-7_9

9.2.2 Superficial Punctate Keratitis

Herpetic viral keratitis is a common manifestation of ocular HSV infection. It can be epithelial, stromal, or endothelial. Epithelial keratitis, characterized by dendritic ulcers, is the hallmark of primary infection. Stromal keratitis involves deeper layers, leading to scarring and potential vision loss. Endothelial involvement, or disciform keratitis, results in stromal edema. Treatment involves topical and systemic antivirals, with corticosteroids used cautiously in stromal disease to reduce inflammation [3, 4].

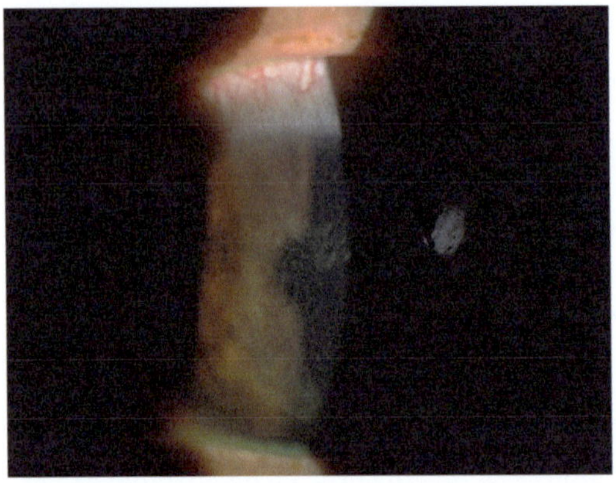

Diffuse illumination slit lamp image depicting superficial punctate keratitis in a patient with herpetic keratitis

9.2.3 Dendritic Keratitis: Fluorescein Staining

Dendritic HSV keratitis is characterized by branching ulcerative lesions on the corneal epithelium. These dendritic ulcers are pathognomonic for HSV infection. Fluorescein staining helps visualize the lesions. Early treatment with topical antiviral medications such as trifluridine or ganciclovir gel is crucial to prevent progression and complications [5].

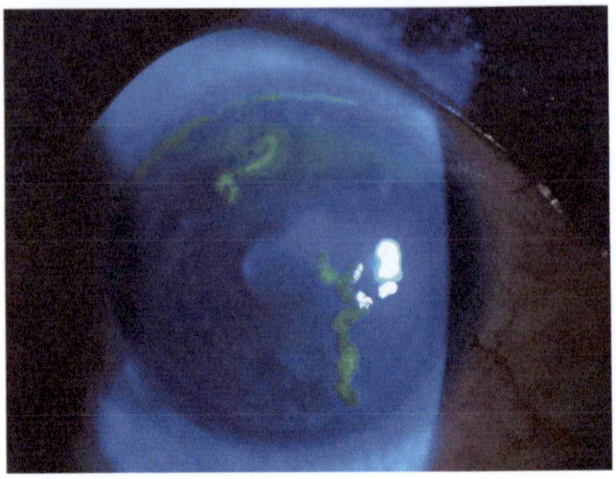

Diffuse illumination slit lamp image of a patient depicting linear dendritic ulcer

9.2.4 Dendritic Keratitis: Rose Bengal Stain

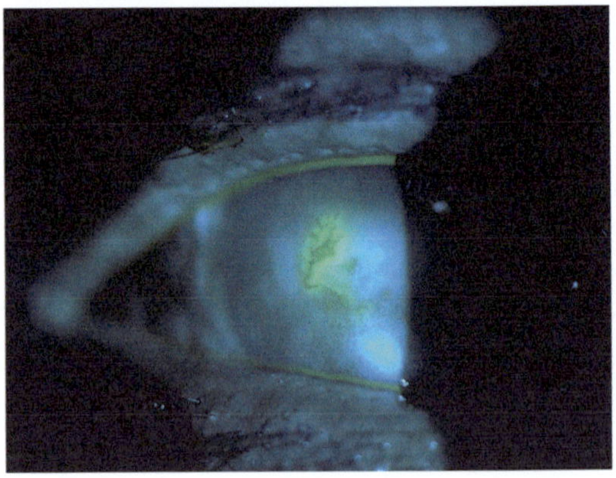

Diffuse illumination slit lamp image of a patient depicting dendritic viral keratitis with fluorescein and Rose Bengal stain

9.2.5 Dendritic Keratitis: Diffuse Image

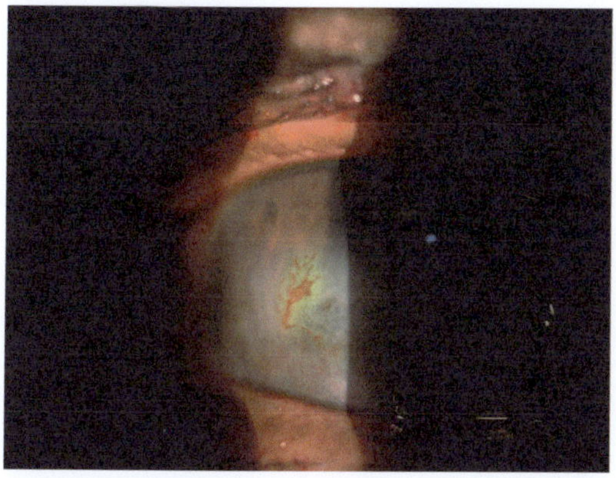

Diffuse illumination slit lamp image of a patient depicting dendritic viral keratitis with fluorescein and Rose Bengal stain

9.2.6 Stromal Keratitis

Viral stromal keratitis involves the deeper layers of the cornea and can result from HSV, varicella-zoster virus (VZV), or other viral pathogens. It is characterized by stromal haze, edema, and potential neovascularization. Corticosteroids and antiviral therapy are the mainstays of treatment, aiming to control inflammation and prevent scarring [6, 7].

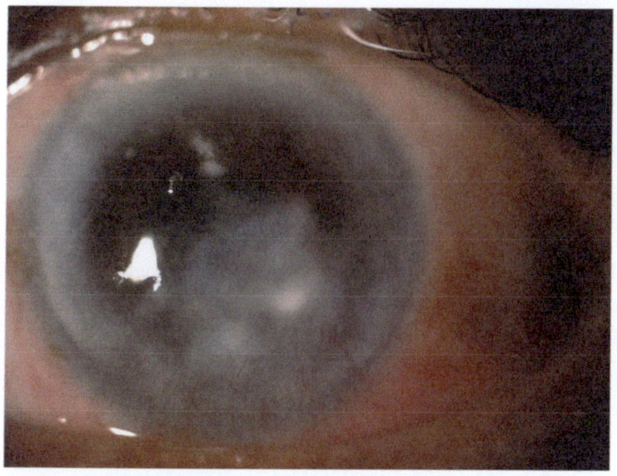

Diffuse illumination slit lamp image depicting stromal infiltrate with superficial and deep vascularization in a patient with viral keratitis

9.2.7 Healed Stromal Keratitis

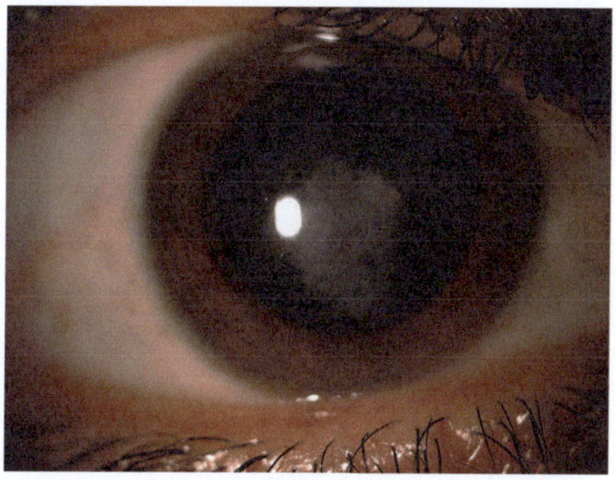

Diffuse illumination slit lamp image of a patient depicting healed viral stromal infiltrate with regressed vessels

9.2.8 Healed Stromal Keratitis

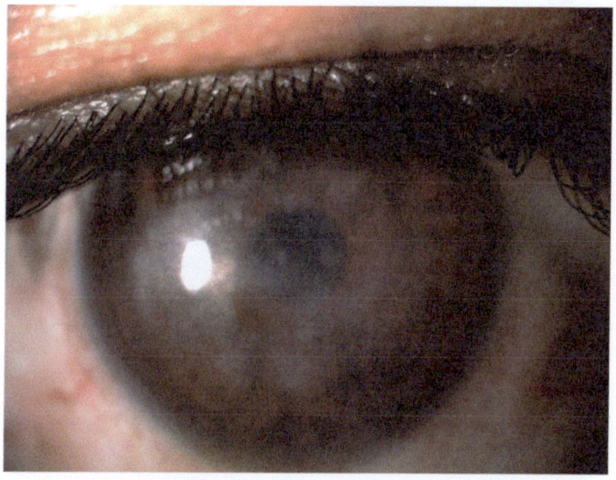

Diffuse illumination slit lamp image of a patient depicting healed viral stromal infiltrate with regressed vessels

9.2.9 Adenoviral Subepithelial Keratitis

Adenoviral keratitis often follows an upper respiratory infection. It can lead to epidemic keratoconjunctivitis, characterized by conjunctival hyperemia, chemosis, and subepithelial infiltrates. These infiltrates can cause prolonged visual disturbances. Management is mainly supportive, including lubricants and cool compresses. In severe cases, topical corticosteroids may be used to reduce subepithelial infiltrates [8, 9].

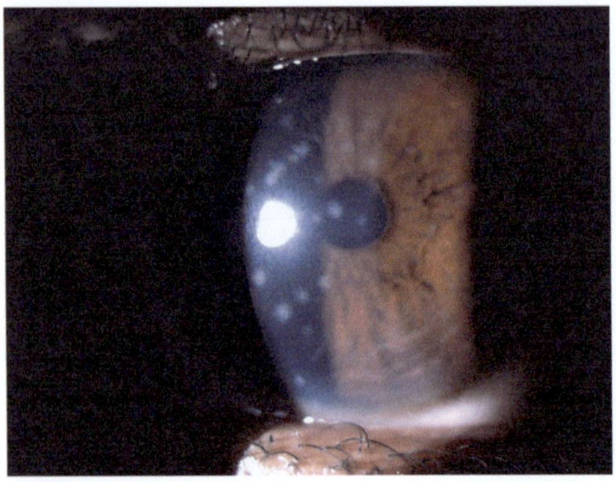

Diffuse illumination slit lamp image of a patient depicting subepithelial active viral keratitis

9.3 Herpes Zoster Virus Manifestations

9.3.1 Conjunctivitis with Stromal Keratitis

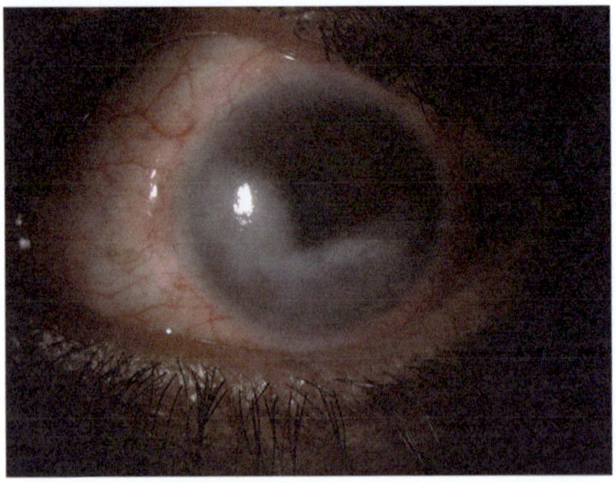

Diffuse illumination slit lamp image depicting stromal infiltrate with superficial and deep vascularization in a patient with viral keratitis

9.3.2 Keratouveitis

Viral keratouveitis is an inflammatory condition involving both the cornea and the uveal tract. It is often associated with HSV or VZV infections. Patients present with pain, photophobia, and decreased vision. Management includes antiviral therapy and corticosteroids to control inflammation and prevent complications like glaucoma or cataract formation [10].

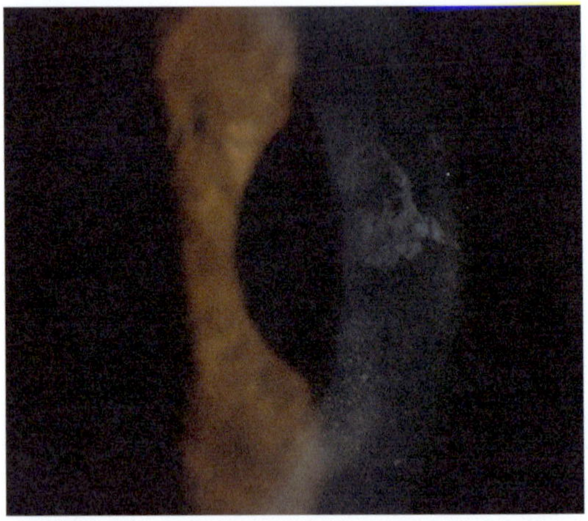

Diffuse illumination slit lamp image of a patient depicting anterior stromal infiltrate with active keratic precipitates suggestive of viral keratouveitis

9.3.3 Keratouveitis

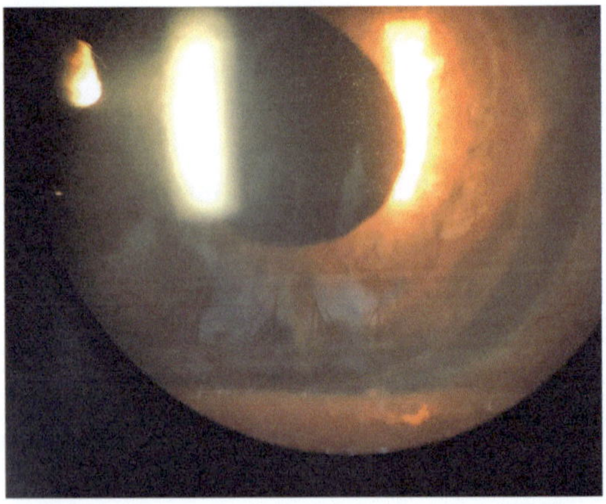

Diffuse illumination slit lamp image of a patient depicting anterior stromal infiltrate with active keratic precipitates and cells in anterior chamber suggestive of viral keratouveitis

9.3.4 Active Nummular Keratitis

Active herpes zoster nummular keratitis occurs in the context of herpes zoster ophthalmicus, a reactivation of VZV. It presents with multiple nummular infiltrates in the corneal stroma, often associated with a vesicular rash. Treatment involves antiviral agents such as oral acyclovir and, in some cases, topical steroids to reduce inflammation [11, 12].

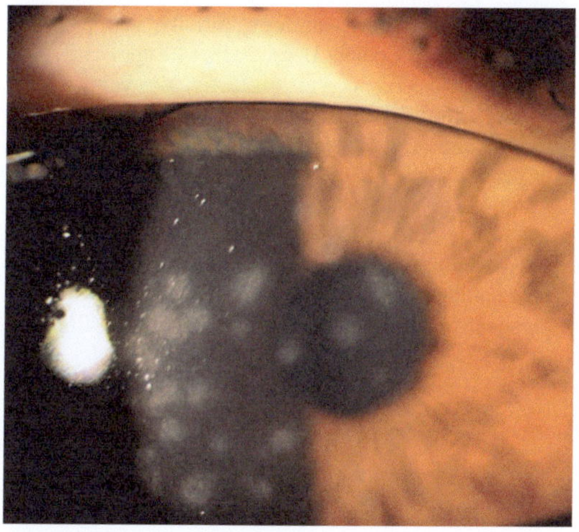

Diffuse illumination slit lamp image of a patient depicting coin-shaped subepithelial and anterior stromal lesions with punctate spots suggestive of viral nummular keratitis

9.3.5 Nummular Scars

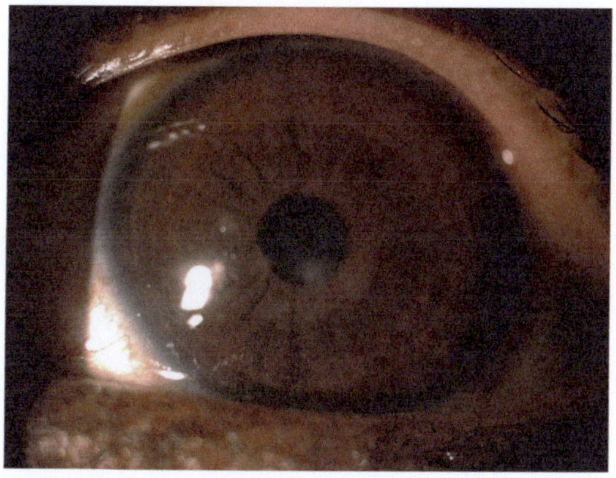

Diffuse illumination slit lamp image of a patient depicting coin-shaped subepithelial scars suggestive of healed viral nummular keratitis

9.3.6 Recurrent Herpes Simplex Keratitis

Recurrent herpes simplex keratitis poses a significant challenge due to its potential for repeated episodes leading to progressive corneal damage. Long-term prophylactic antiviral therapy can reduce recurrence rates. Each episode requires prompt antiviral treatment to minimize complications and preserve corneal integrity [4].

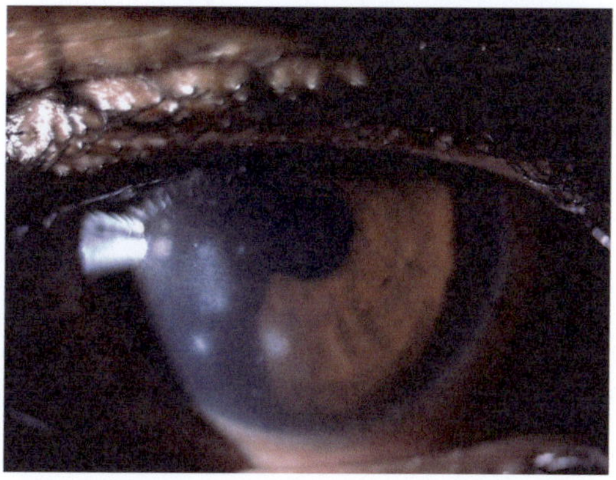

Diffuse illumination slit lamp image of a patient depicting active subepithelial infiltrates suggestive of recurrent herpes simplex keratitis

9.3.7 Viral Keratitis with Secondary Bacterial Infiltrate

Viral keratitis with secondary bacterial infiltrate occurs when a bacterial infection supervenes on a viral corneal lesion. This condition is more severe and requires combined antiviral and antibacterial therapy. Prompt recognition and treatment are crucial to prevent corneal perforation and vision loss [13].

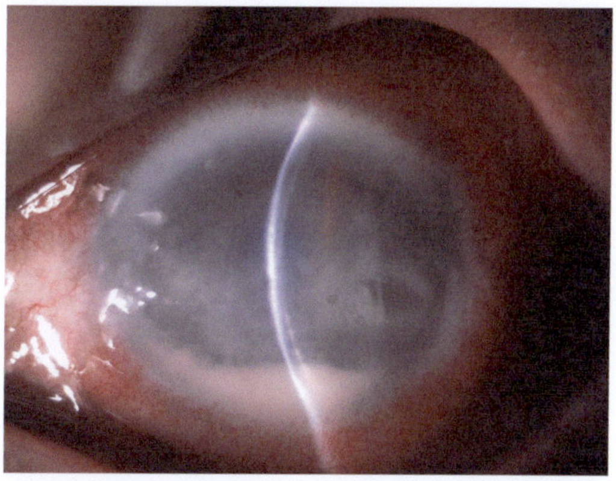

Diffuse illumination slit lamp image of a patient depicting temporal epithelial defect with anterior stromal infiltrate with a hypopyon

References

1. Kaye S, Choudhary A. Herpes simplex keratitis. Prog Retin Eye Res. 2006;25(4):355–80.
2. Liesegang TJ. Herpes simplex virus epidemiology and ocular importance. Cornea. 2001;20(1):1–13.
3. Farooq AV, Shukla D. Herpes simplex epithelial and stromal keratitis: an epidemiologic update. Surv Ophthalmol. 2012;57(5):448–62.
4. Wilhelmus KR. Therapeutic interventions for herpes simplex virus epithelial keratitis. Cochrane Database Syst Rev. 2010;12:CD002898.
5. Labetoulle M, et al. Expert consensus on the management of herpes simplex virus keratitis: a modified Delphi panel approach. Br J Ophthalmol. 2017;101(5):622–7.
6. Kaye SB, et al. Antiviral therapy for herpes simplex virus (HSV) keratitis: a systematic review and meta-analysis. Ocul Surf. 2020;18(4):688–99.
7. Toma HS, et al. Ocular HSV-1 latency, reactivation, and recurrent disease. Exp Eye Res. 2008;87(5):454–65.
8. Jhanji V, et al. Adenoviral keratitis. Curr Opin Ophthalmol. 2013;24(4):403–9.
9. García-Zalisnak D, et al. Adenovirus ocular infections: prevalence, pathology, pitfalls, and practical pointers. Eye Contact Lens. 2018;44(Suppl 1):S1–7.
10. Miserocchi E, et al. Infectious uveitis. Dev Ophthalmol. 2012;51:148–62.
11. Liesegang TJ. Varicella zoster virus eye disease. Cornea. 1999;18(5):511–31.
12. Tran KD, et al. Herpes zoster ophthalmicus. Curr Ophthalmol Rep. 2014;2:174–9.
13. Kaye S, et al. Antibacterial and antiviral therapy in the management of bacterial keratitis and viral keratitis, respectively. Am J Ophthalmol. 2012;154(2):268–74.

10 Bacterial, Fungal, and Parasitic Infectious Diseases of the Cornea and External Eye

Radhika Natarajan, Madhuvanthi Mohan, Bharat Gurnani, and Kirandeep Kaur

10.1 Introduction

Infectious keratitis is a critical ophthalmic condition characterized by the invasion of the cornea by various pathogens, leading to corneal inflammation and ulceration. It can result in significant visual impairment and blindness if not promptly treated. This introduction discusses several types of infectious keratitis, including bacterial, fungal, acanthamoeba, and others, highlighting their clinical features, diagnostic modalities, and management strategies.

10.2 Bacterial Corneal Ulcer

10.2.1 Corneal Melt with Hypopyon

Bacterial corneal ulcers are a common cause of infectious keratitis, often resulting from trauma, contact lens wear, or pre-existing ocular surface disease. Common pathogens include *Staphylococcus aureus*, *Pseudomonas aeruginosa*, and *Streptococcus pneumoniae*. Clinical presentation includes pain, redness, discharge, and a central or paracentral corneal ulcer. Diagnosis is confirmed by corneal scraping and culture. Treatment involves broad-spectrum topical antibiotics, adjusted based on culture results [1, 2].

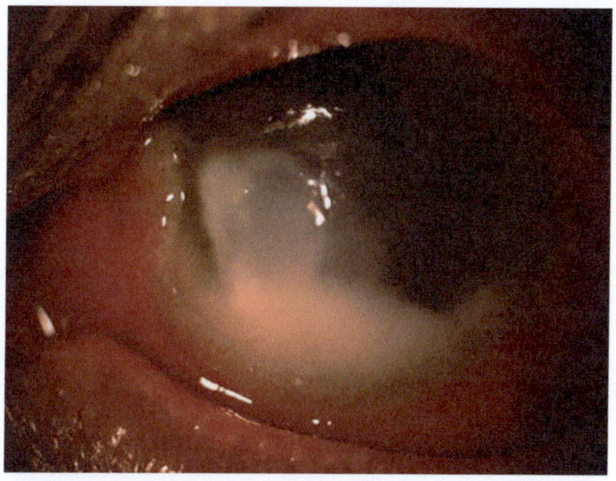

Diffuse illumination slit lamp image of a patient with Staphylococcal bacterial keratitis depicting anterior to mid-stromal infiltrate with a hypopyon

R. Natarajan (✉) · M. Mohan
Department of Cornea and Refractive Surgery, Sankara Netralaya Medical Research Foundation, Chennai, Tamil Nadu, India
e-mail: drnr@snmail.org

B. Gurnani
Department of Cataract, Cornea, Trauma, External Diseases, Ocular Surface and Refractive Services, Gomabai Netralaya and Research Centre, Neemuch, Madhya Pradesh, India

K. Kaur
Department of Cataract, Pediatric Ophthalmology and Strabismus, Gomabai Netralaya and Research Centre, Neemuch, Madhya Pradesh, India

B. Gurnani, K. Kaur (eds.), *Atlas of Cornea*, https://doi.org/10.1007/978-981-96-0013-7_10

10.2.2 Ring Infiltrate with Hypopyon

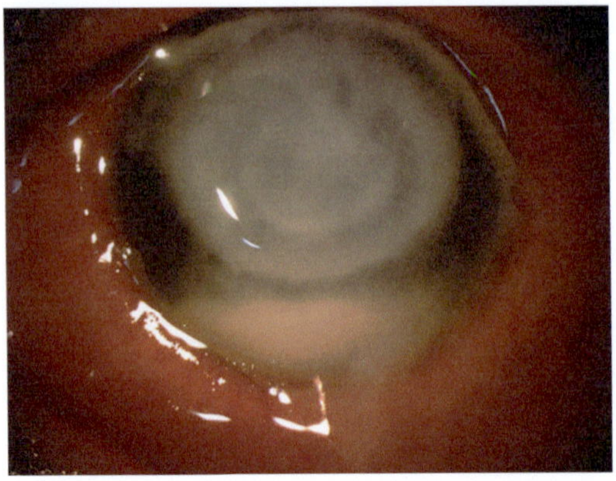

Diffuse illumination slit lamp image of a patient with Pseudomonas keratitis depicting full-thickness ring corneal infiltrate with a hypopyon

10.2.3 Healed Pseudomonas Keratitis

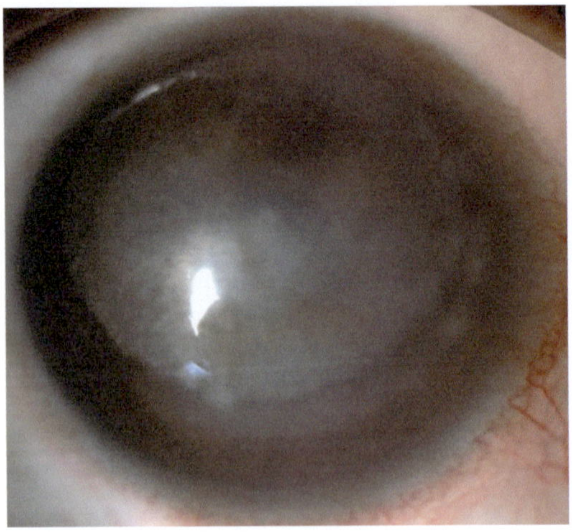

Diffuse illumination slit lamp image of a patient depicting healed Pseudomonas keratitis with a nebulomacular corneal scar

10.3 Fungal Keratitis

10.3.1 Central Corneal Infiltrate with Thinning

Fungal keratitis, caused by filamentous fungi (e.g., Fusarium, Aspergillus) or yeast (e.g., Candida), is more common in tropical climates and agricultural workers. Symptoms include pain, photophobia, and discharge, with characteristic feathery infiltrates or raised ulcers. Diagnosis is achieved through corneal scraping, culture, and histopathology. Antifungal therapy with agents like natamycin or voriconazole is the mainstay of treatment, but surgical intervention may be necessary in advanced cases [3, 4].

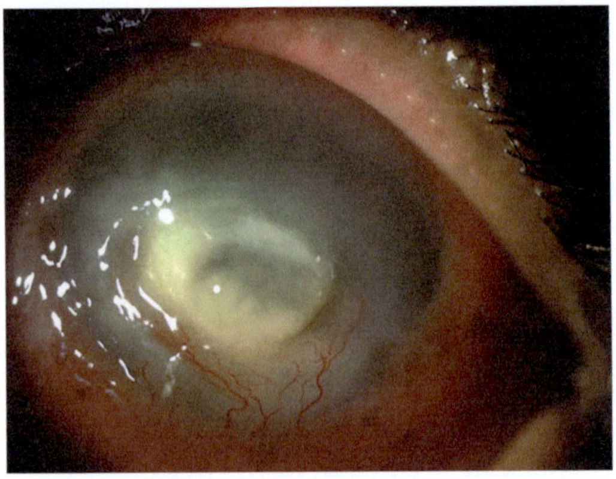

Diffuse illumination slit lamp image of a patient depicting full-thickness central corneal infiltrate with thinning and superficial corneal vascularization in a patient with fungal keratitis

10.3.2 Deep Mycosis

Deep fungal keratitis is a severe infection of the corneal stroma caused by fungi such as Fusarium and Aspergillus species. This condition often presents with pain, redness, and reduced vision and requires aggressive antifungal therapy and sometimes surgical intervention to prevent progression and preserve vision [5].

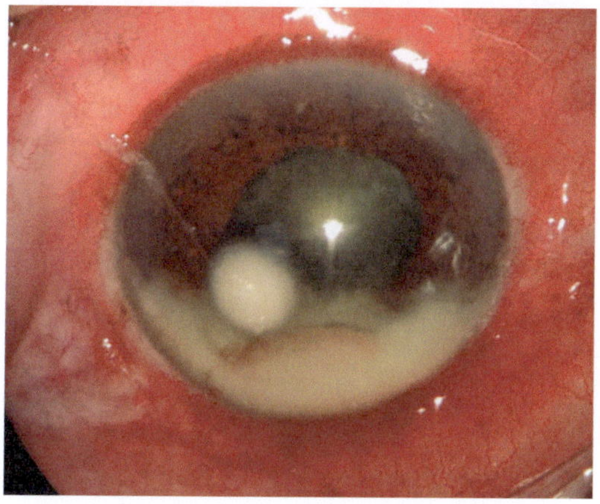

Diffuse illumination slit lamp image depicting 2 × 3 mm full-thickness circular corneal ulcer (deep mycosis) with large hypopyon in a patient with fungal keratitis

10.3.3 Dematiaceous Fungal Keratitis

Dematiaceous fungal keratitis, caused by pigmented fungi like Exserohilum and Curvularia, presents with pigmented corneal infiltrates. These infections are particularly challenging due to their resistance to conventional antifungal agents. Diagnosis relies on microbiological and histopathological evaluation, and treatment often requires a combination of medical and surgical approaches [6].

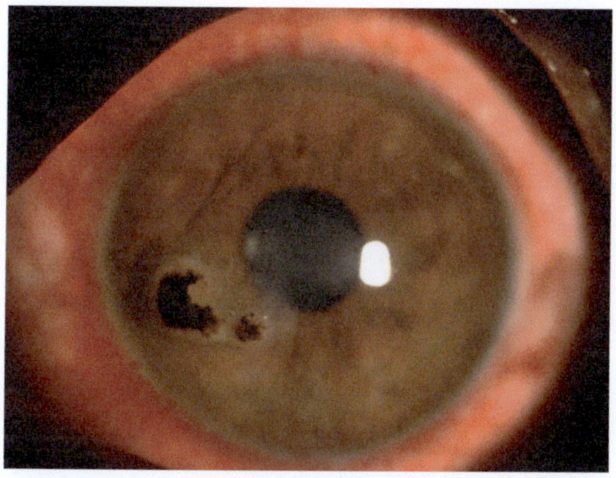

Diffuse illumination slit lamp image depicting paralimbal pigmented corneal infiltrate in a patient with fungal keratitis

10.3.4 Posterior Stromal Infiltrate

Fungal keratitis with hypopyon is a severe corneal infection characterized by fungal infiltration and the presence of inflammatory cells in the anterior chamber. This condition often presents with pain, decreased vision, and a visible white or yellowish layer of pus in the anterior chamber, requiring prompt antifungal treatment and possibly surgical intervention to prevent further complications and preserve vision [7].

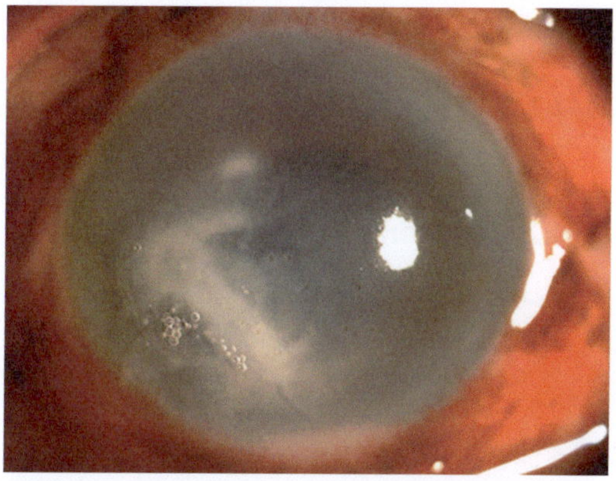

Diffuse illumination slit lamp image depicting irregularly-shaped 5 × 3 mm mid-to-posterior stromal corneal ulcer with streak hypopyon in a patient with fungal keratitis

10.4 Acanthamoeba Keratitis

10.4.1 Ring Infiltrate

Acanthamoeba keratitis is associated with contact lens misuse and exposure to contaminated water. It presents with severe pain, ring infiltrates, and radial keratoneuritis. Diagnosis is challenging and often delayed, requiring corneal scrapings, confocal microscopy, and culture. Treatment includes topical anti-amoebic agents like polyhexamethylene biguanide (PHMB) and chlorhexidine, but prolonged therapy is often needed [8, 9].

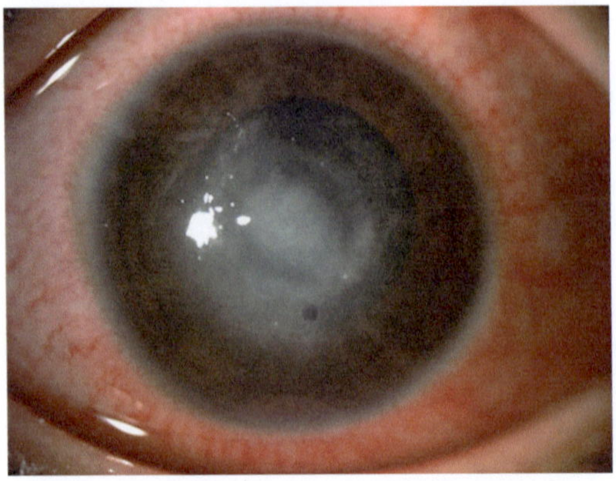

Diffuse illumination slit lamp image depicting central ring-shaped corneal infiltrate in a patient with Acanthamoeba keratitis

10.4.2 Resolving Keratitis

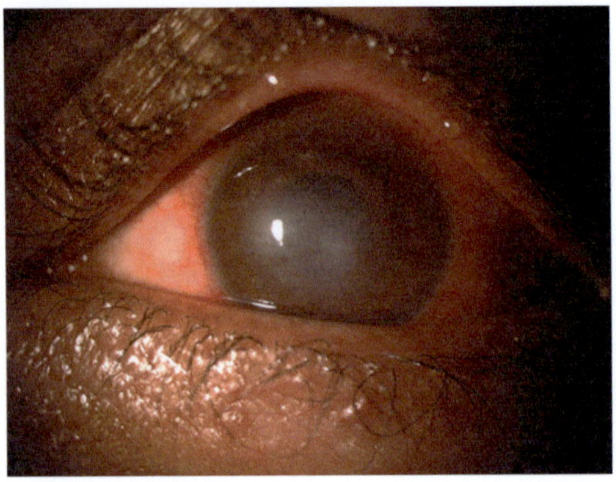

Diffuse illumination slit lamp image depicting anterior stromal haze with healed infiltrate in a patient with Acanthamoeba keratitis

10.5 Pythium Insidiosum Keratitis

10.5.1 Early and Total Corneal Infiltrate

Pythium insidiosum keratitis, a rare but severe infection, mimics fungal keratitis. It typically affects individuals in tropical regions. Clinical features include necrotizing lesions and a poor response to antifungal therapy. Diagnosis is confirmed through culture and molecular methods. Treatment is challenging, often requiring aggressive surgical intervention [10, 11].

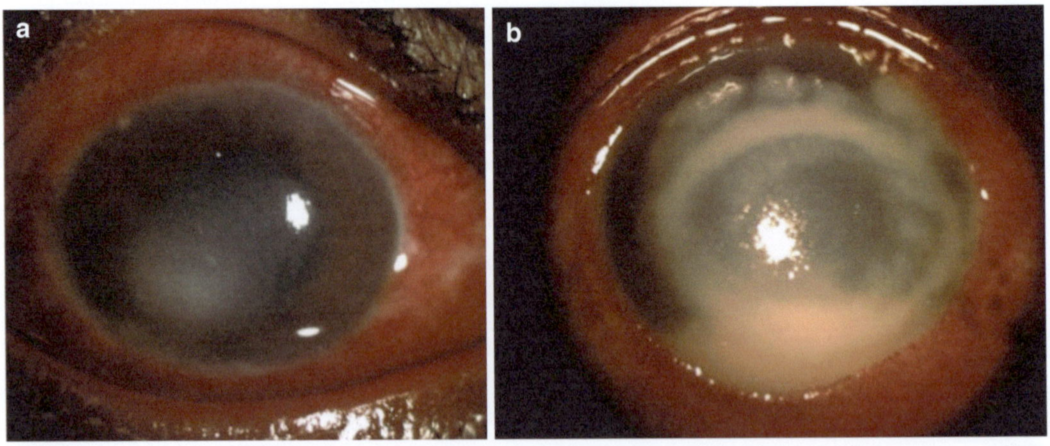

Diffuse illumination slit lamp image depicting (**a**) inferior paracentral anterior stromal infiltrate with streak hypopyon and (**b**) total full-thickness ring-shaped corneal infiltrate with early limbal spread and hypopyon

10.5.2 Tentacular Projections

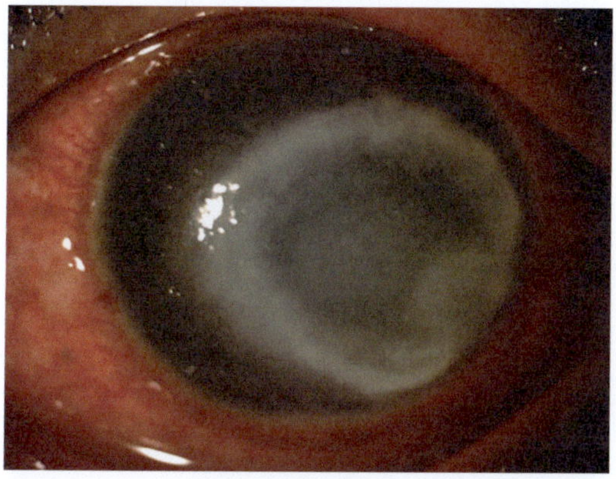

Diffuse illumination slit lamp image of a patient depicting full-thickness corneal infiltrate with tentacular projections

10.6 Contact Lens-Induced Keratitis (CLIK)

10.6.1 Central Corneal Infiltrate with Hypopyon

Contact lens-induced keratitis is a significant risk for contact lens wearers, often due to poor hygiene practices. It can be bacterial, fungal, or amoebic. Prevention through education on proper lens care is crucial, and treatment involves appropriate antimicrobial therapy based on the identified pathogen [12].

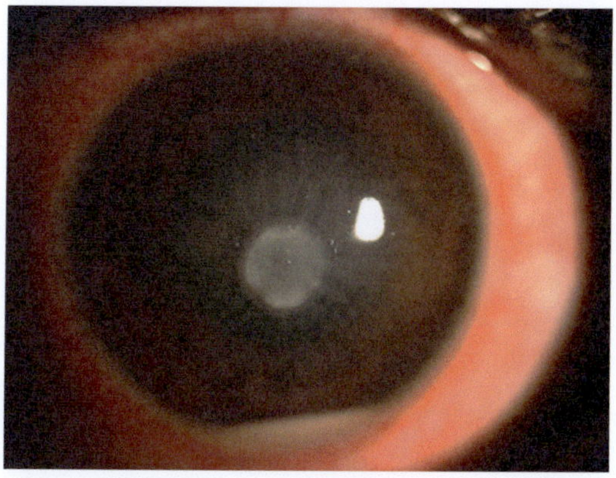

Diffuse illumination slit lamp image of a patient depicting 2x2 mm central corneal ulcer and descemet membrane folds with streak hypopyon in a regular contact lens wearer

10.6.2 Healing CLIK

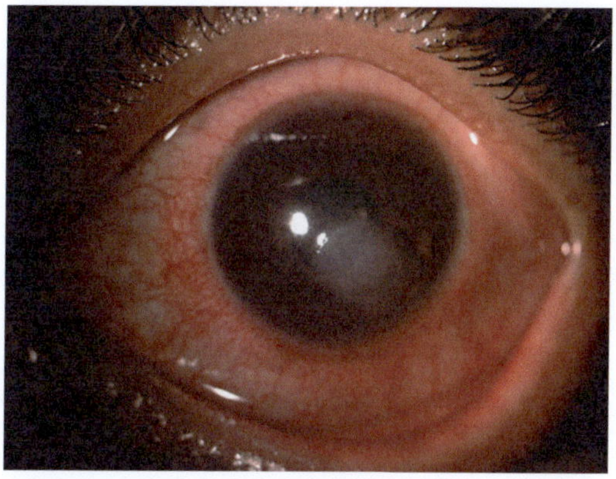

Diffuse illumination slit lamp image of a patient depicting healing paracentral corneal ulcer in a regular contact lens wearer

10.6.3 Healed CL Keratitis

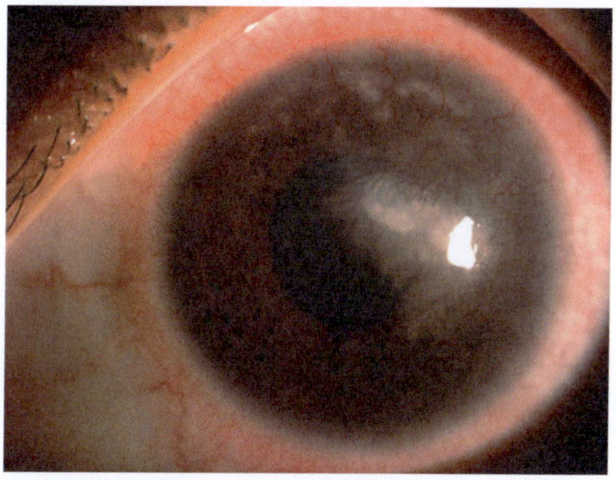

Diffuse illumination slit lamp image of a patient depicting healed corneal ulcer with anterior stromal scarring and superficial vascularization in a regular contact lens wearer

10.6.4 Healed CL Keratitis

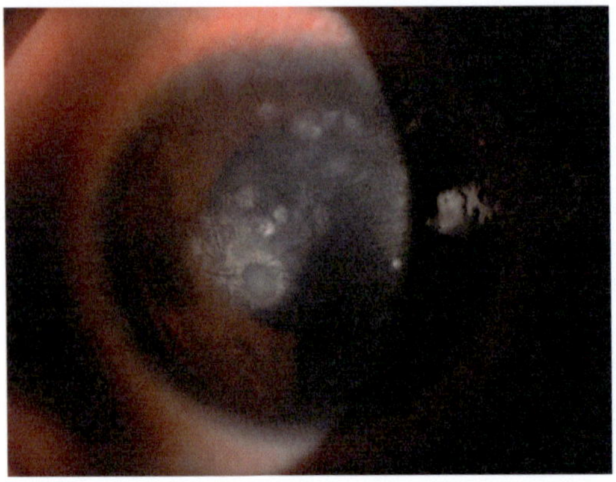

Diffuse illumination slit lamp image of a patient depicting healed corneal ulcer with anterior stromal scarring and superficial vascularization in a regular contact lens wearer

10.6.5 Atypical Mycobacterial Keratitis

Atypical mycobacterial keratitis, caused by organisms like *Mycobacterium chelonae*, presents with chronic, indolent ulcers. Diagnosis requires specialized culture techniques and PCR. Treatment includes prolonged antibiotic therapy with agents like clarithromycin and amikacin, often necessitating adjunctive surgical intervention [13, 14].

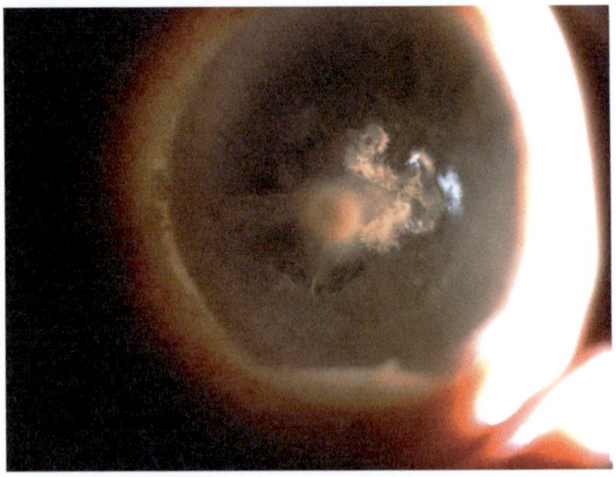

Diffuse illumination slit lamp image of a patient depicting central active midstromal infiltrate with surrounding corneal scar and hypopyon

10.6.6 Anterior Segment Optical Coherence Tomography in Atypical Mycobacterial Keratitis

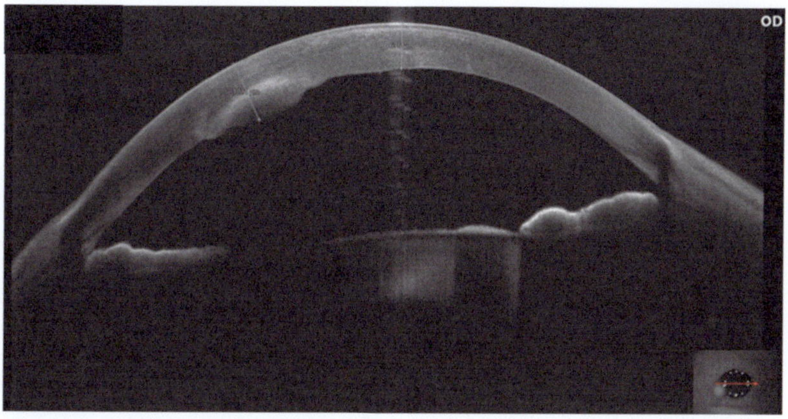

Anterior segment optical coherence tomography showing deep stromal involvement in a patient with atypical mycobacterial keratitis

10.7 Microsporidial Keratitis

10.7.1 Punctate Epithelial Keratitis

Microsporidial keratitis, caused by obligate intracellular parasites, often affects immunocompromised individuals. It presents with multiple punctate epithelial lesions. Diagnosis is confirmed through light microscopy and PCR. Treatment options are limited, with topical fumagillin showing some efficacy [15].

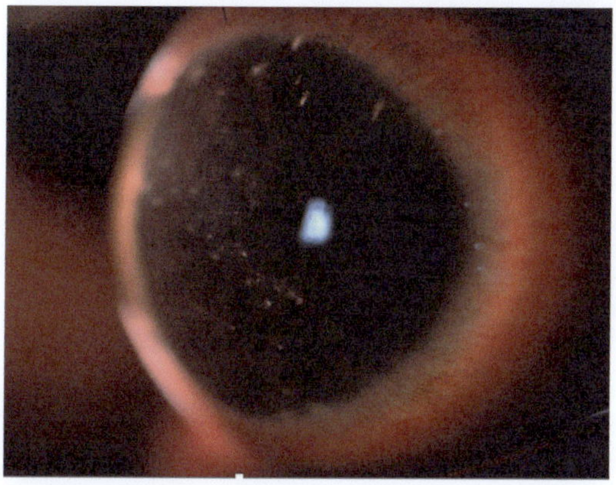

Diffuse illumination slit lamp image depicting punctate epithelial keratitis with the characteristic stuck-on appearance in a patient with microsporidial keratitis

10.7.2 Coarse Superficial Punctate Epithelial Keratitis

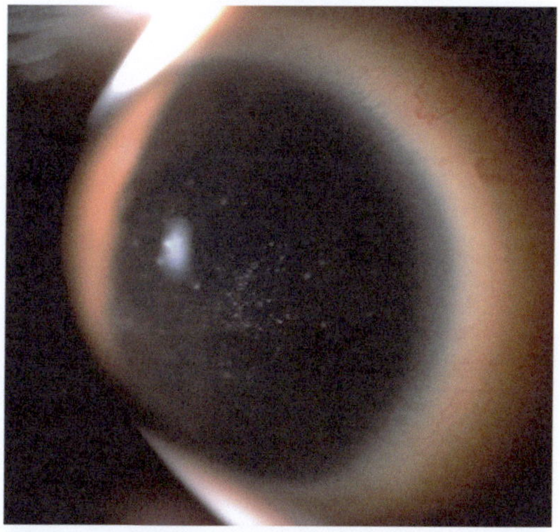

Diffuse illumination slit lamp image depicting punctate epithelial keratitis with the characteristic stuck-on appearance in a patient with microsporidial keratitis

10.7.3 Fluorescein-Stained Superficial Punctate Epithelial Keratitis

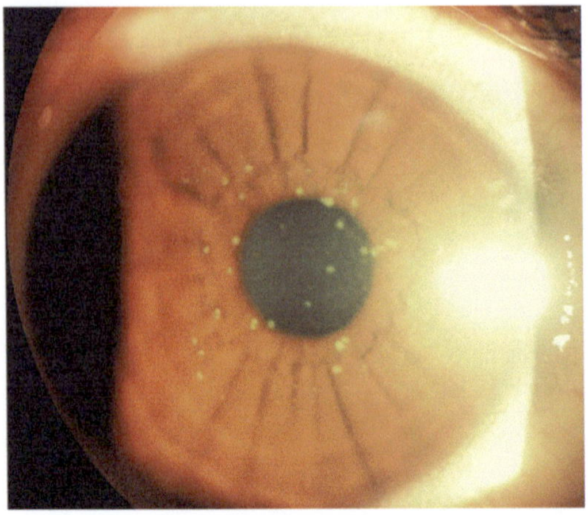

Diffuse illumination slit lamp image of a patient depicting fluorescein-stained punctate epithelial keratitis with the characteristic stuck-on appearance in a patient with microsporidial keratitis

10.7.4 Infectious Keratitis Post-Manual Small-Incision Cataract Surgery

Post-surgical infectious keratitis, particularly following manual small-incision cataract surgery, poses a significant threat. It necessitates prompt identification of the causative organism and aggressive antimicrobial therapy to prevent complications [16].

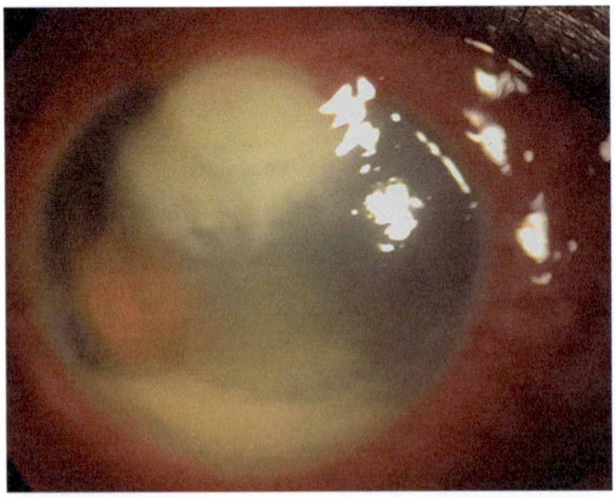

Diffuse illumination slit lamp image depicting total corneal infiltrate along the superior cornea involving the surgical section with hypopyon in a patient post-manual small-incision cataract surgery

10.8 Graft Infection

10.8.1 Ring Infiltrate

Graft infection is a serious complication following corneal transplantation. It requires intensive antimicrobial treatment and, in some cases, surgical revision to preserve the graft integrity and function [17, 18].

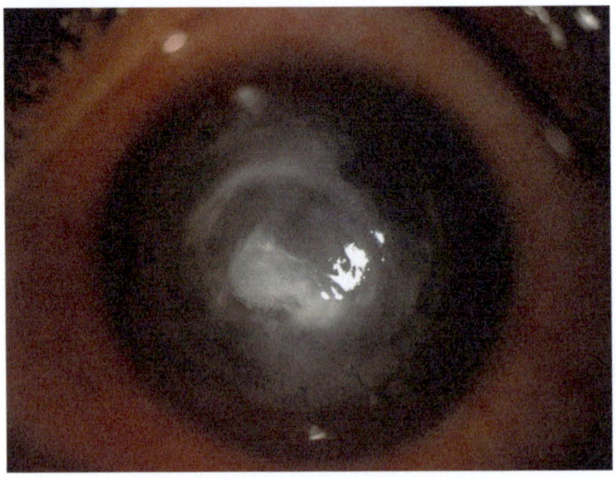

Diffuse illumination slit lamp image of a patient depicting anterior-to-mid-stromal infiltrate post-optical penetrating keratoplasty

10.8.2 Corneal Infiltrate with Hypopyon

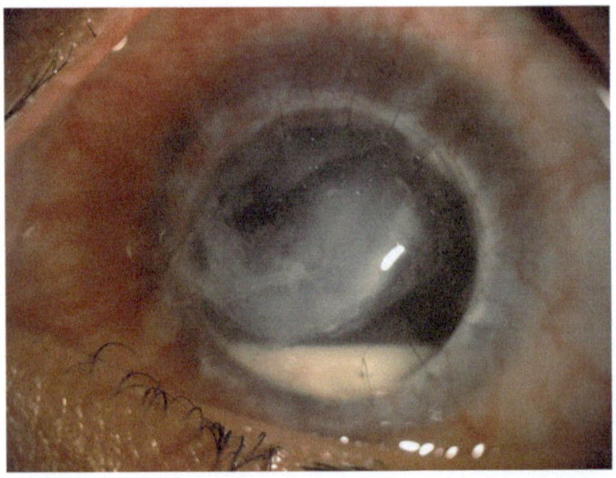

Diffuse illumination slit lamp image of a patient depicting anterior-to-mid-stromal infiltrate (bacterial) with hypopyon suggestive of graft infection post-optical penetrating keratoplasty

10.9 Peripheral Ulcerative Keratitis

10.9.1 Guttering with Infiltration

Peripheral ulcerative keratitis (PUK) with infiltration is a severe corneal condition characterized by peripheral corneal thinning, ulceration, and infiltration by inflammatory cells. It is often associated with systemic autoimmune diseases like rheumatoid arthritis, necessitating aggressive management with topical and systemic immunosuppressive therapies to control the inflammation and prevent further corneal damage [19].

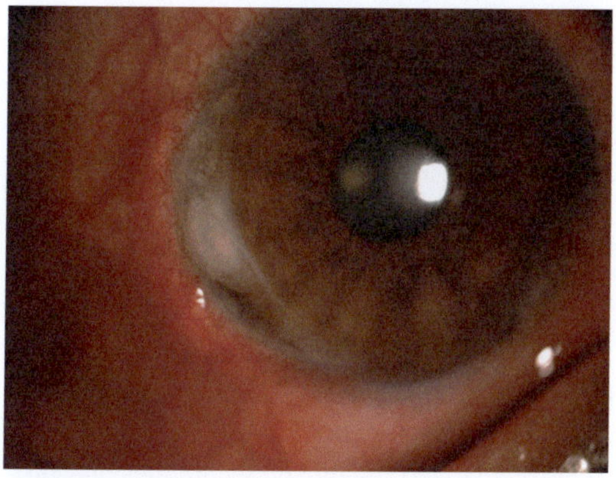

Diffuse illumination slit lamp image depicting temporal crescent-shaped anterior-to-mid-stromal infiltrate (bacterial) along the limbus with guttering in a peripheral ulcerative keratitis patient

10.9.2 Limbal Guttering with Thinning

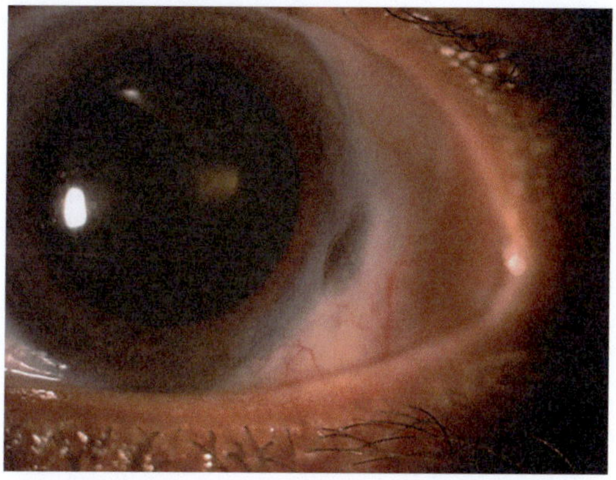

Diffuse illumination slit lamp image depicting a nasal crescent-shaped stromal infiltrate along the limbus with guttering in a peripheral ulcerative keratitis patient

10.10 Descemetocele in a

10.10.1 Failed Graft

Descemetocele formation, a severe complication in various types of keratitis (bacterial, fungal, and sterile), indicates deep stromal involvement and an imminent risk of perforation. Management includes aggressive antimicrobial therapy and surgical interventions such as tissue adhesive application or keratoplasty [20, 21].

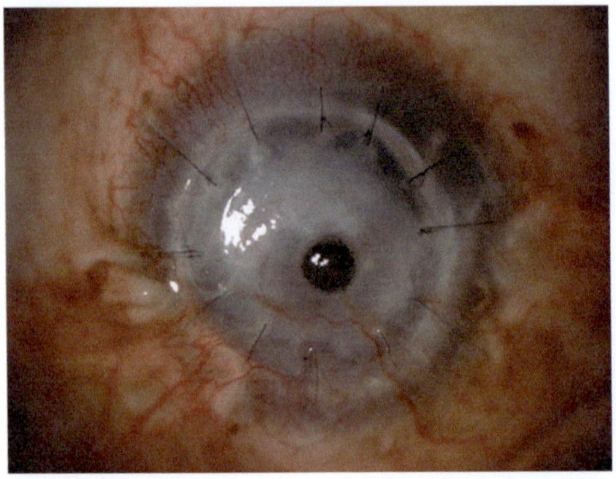

Diffuse illumination slit lamp image of a patient depicting Central descemetocele in a failed corneal graft with superficial and deep vascularization

10.10.2 Fungal Keratitis

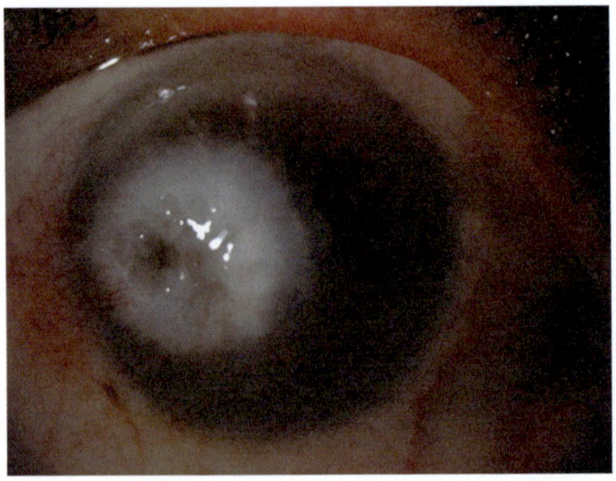

Diffuse illumination slit lamp image of a patient depicting 5 × 5 mm paracentral leukomatous corneal scar with descemetocele in a patient with fungal keratitis

10.10.3 Sterile Corneal Ulcer

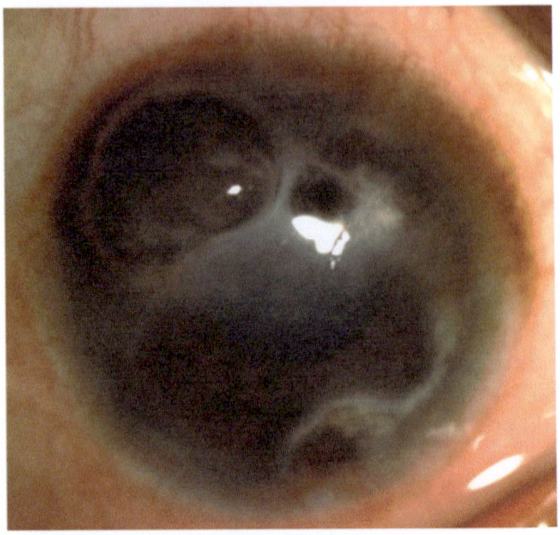

Diffuse illumination slit lamp image of a patient depicting superior and inferior corneal thinning with descemetocele in a patient with sterile corneal infiltrate

10.10.4 Nocardia Keratitis

Nocardia keratitis and pigmented fungal keratitis are rare but challenging infections. They necessitate specialized diagnostic techniques and prolonged antimicrobial therapy [22, 23].

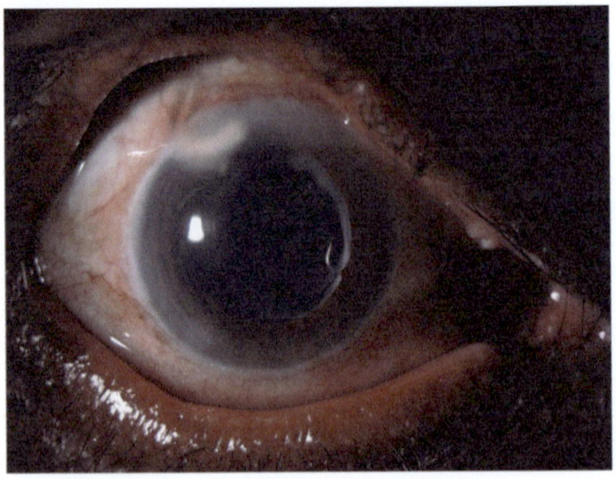

Diffuse illumination slit lamp image of a patient depicting full-thickness corneal infiltrate in the superior cornea suggestive of Nocardia keratitis

10.10.5 Therapeutic Corneal Scraping in Infectious Keratitis

Therapeutic corneal scraping is a valuable adjunctive procedure in managing infectious keratitis, facilitating pathogen identification and enhancing antimicrobial penetration [24].

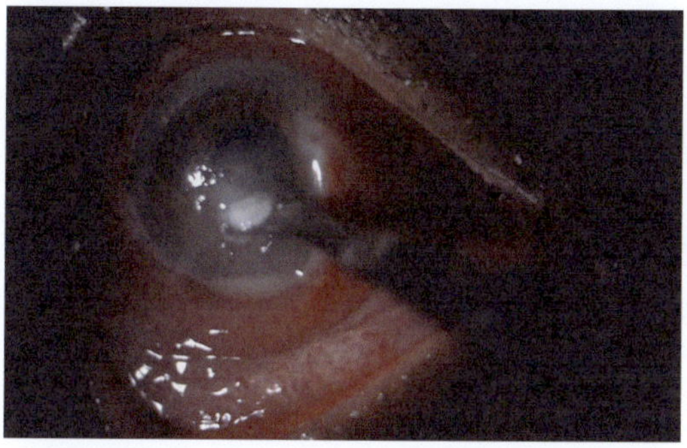

Diffuse illumination slit lamp image of a patient depicting corneal scraping being performed for superficial corneal ulcer with a Bard Parker blade

10.11 Pigmented Fungal Corneal Ulcer

10.11.1 Nasal Corneal Infiltrate

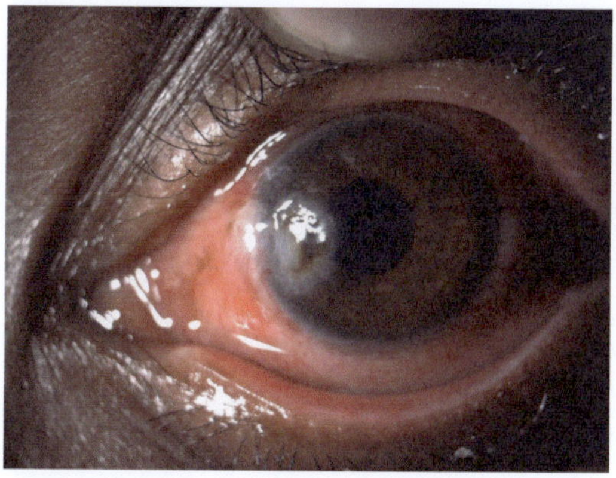

Diffuse illumination slit lamp image depicting a temporal pigmented anterior stromal infiltrate with thinning with pigmentation in a patient with fungal corneal ulcer

10.12 Pigmented Fungal Corneal Ulcer

10.12.1 Corneal Infiltrate with Hypopyon

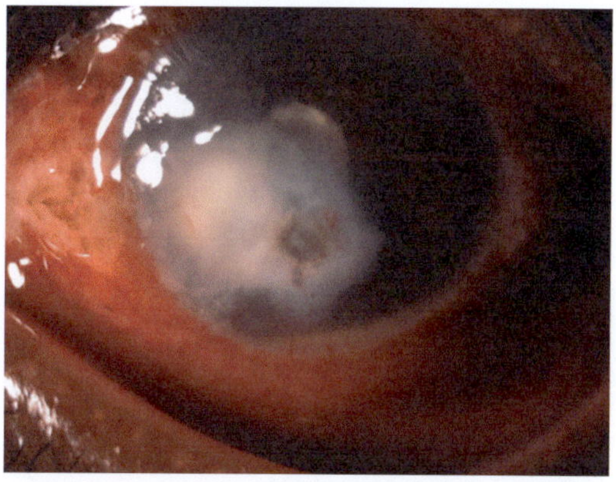

Diffuse illumination slit lamp image depicting full-thickness corneal infiltrate with pigmentation with hypopyon in a patient with fungal corneal ulcer

10.12.2 Post-DALK Infectious Keratitis

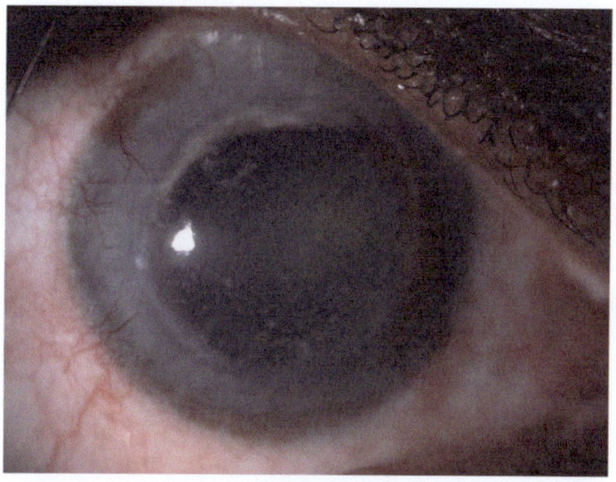

Diffuse illumination slit lamp image depicting active corneal infiltration at the graft host junction in a patient post-DALK

10.13 Infectious Crystalline Keratopathy

10.13.1 Central Epithelial Defect with Corneal Infiltrate

Infectious crystalline keratopathy, typically caused by *Streptococcus viridans*, presents with branching crystalline infiltrates. Diagnosis relies on clinical examination and microbiological studies, and treatment involves targeted antibiotic therapy [25].

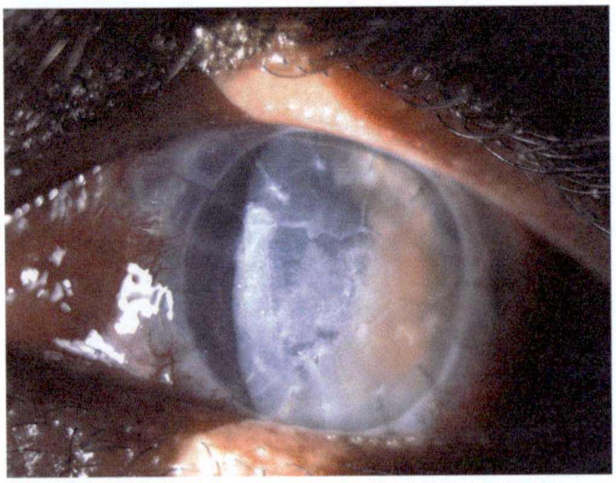

Diffuse illumination slit lamp image depicting central epithelial defect with anterior stromal infiltrate in a patient post-optical penetrating keratoplasty

10.13.2 Focal Plaque-Like Corneal Infiltrate

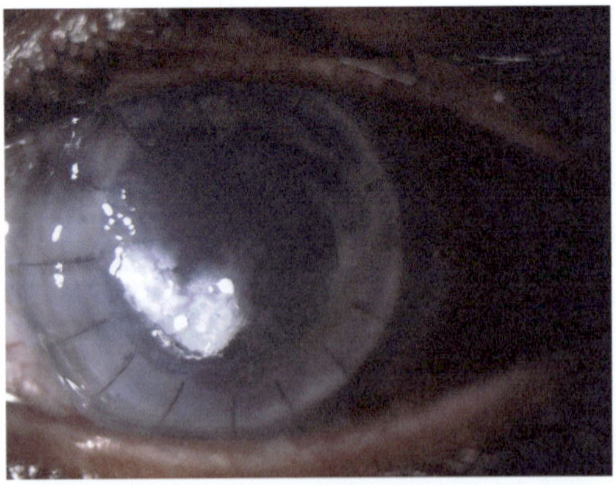

Diffuse illumination slit lamp image depicting silvery crystalline anterior stromal infiltrate in a patient post-optical penetrating keratoplasty

10.13.3 Gram-Negative Bacilli: Bacterial Keratitis

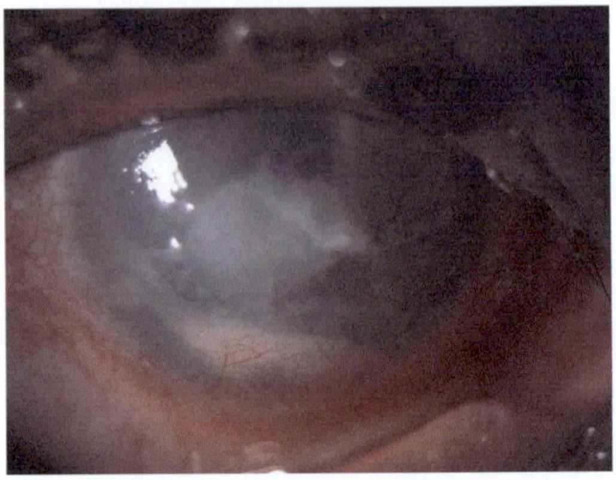

Diffuse illumination slit lamp image of a patient depicting central anterior stromal infiltrate with hypopyon and superficial vascularization inferiorly

10.13.4 Post-Descemet Stripping Endothelial Keratoplasty Fungal Keratitis

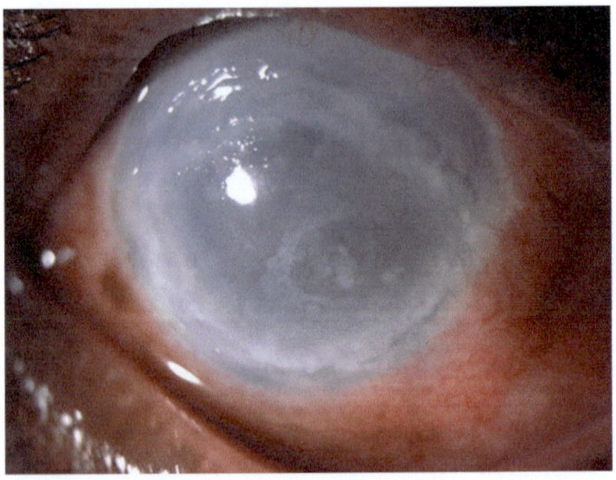

Diffuse illumination slit lamp image depicting paracentral epithelial defect with total corneal ulcer in a patient post-Descemet stripping endothelial keratoplasty

10.13.5 Large Epithelial Defect

An epithelial defect in the cornea is characterized by the loss of the corneal epithelium, which can result from trauma, infection, or underlying ocular surface disease. Such defects can cause pain, tearing, and potential vision loss, requiring prompt management with lubricants, bandage contact lenses, and sometimes surgical interventions to promote re-epithelialization and prevent complications [26].

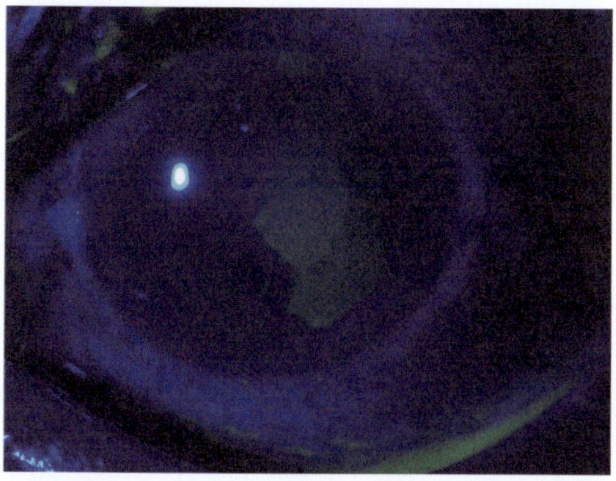

Diffuse illumination slit lamp image of a patient depicting large epithelial defects with fluorescein staining under cobalt blue filter

10.13.6 Perforated Corneal Ulcer: Post-Glue and BCL

A perforated corneal ulcer is a serious condition where the corneal tissue is severely compromised, leading to a full-thickness defect. After the application of tissue adhesive (glue) and a bandage contact lens (BCL), the aim is to seal the perforation, promote re-epithelialization, and stabilize the cornea, thereby preventing further complications such as endophthalmitis and promoting healing [27].

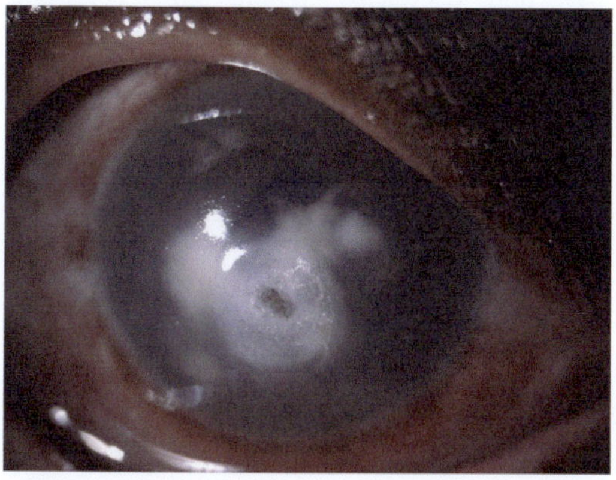

Diffuse illumination slit lamp image of a patient depicting central corneal infiltrate with perforation and glue plaque sealing the perforation

10.13.7 Gram-Positive Cocci Keratitis

Gram-positive cocci keratitis is a bacterial infection of the cornea caused by organisms such as Staphylococcus and Streptococcus species. It presents with symptoms like pain, redness, and decreased vision and requires prompt antibiotic therapy to eradicate the infection and prevent complications such as corneal perforation [28].

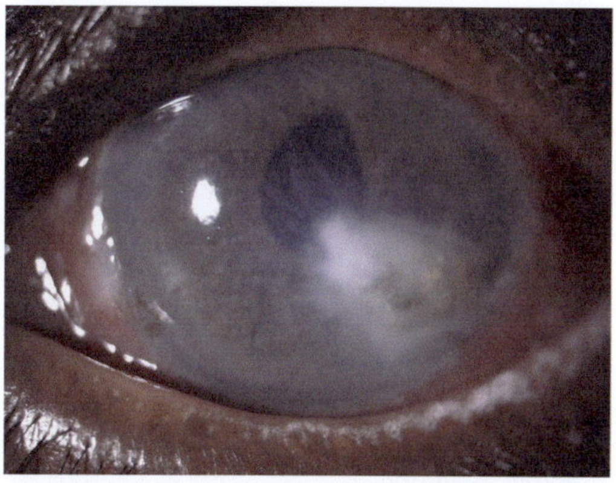

Diffuse illumination slit lamp image of a patient depicting paracentral anterior-to-midstromal corneal infiltrate with Descemet membrane folds and climatic droplet keratopathy

10.13.8 Pythium Insidiosum Keratitis with Corneal Melt

Pythium insidiosum keratitis is a rare and aggressive infection of the cornea that can lead to severe inflammation and corneal melt. It is characterized by rapid progression and poor response to conventional antifungal therapy, often necessitating surgical interventions such as corneal transplantation to prevent vision loss and restore ocular integrity [29].

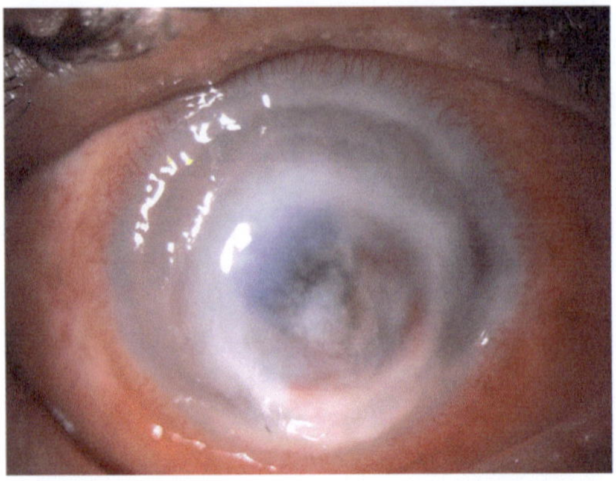

Diffuse illumination slit lamp image depicting total corneal infiltrate with central thinning and stromal melt in a patient with Pythium insidiosum keratitis

10.13.9 Staphylococcal Corneal Abscess

Staphylococcal corneal abscess is a localized bacterial infection of the cornea caused by Staphylococcus species. It presents with symptoms such as severe pain, redness, and visual impairment. Management involves prompt antibiotic therapy to eradicate the infection and prevent complications such as corneal perforation and scarring [30].

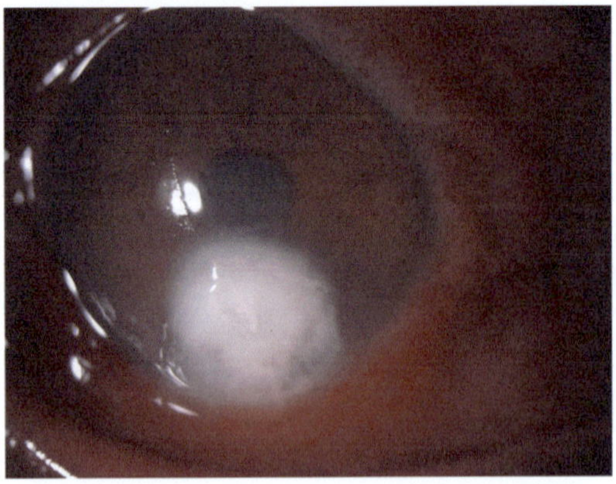

Diffuse illumination slit lamp image of a patient depicting inferior full-thickness corneal infiltrate suggestive of staphylococcal abscess

10.13.10 Exserohilum Keratitis

Exserohilum keratitis is a rare fungal infection of the cornea caused by Exserohilum species. It typically presents with symptoms like pain, redness, and decreased vision. Due to its aggressive nature and poor response to conventional antifungal therapy, early diagnosis and prompt treatment, including surgical intervention, are critical to prevent severe complications and preserve vision [31].

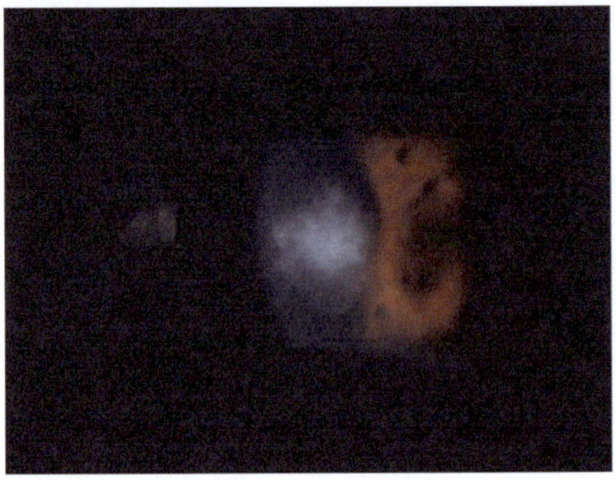

Diffuse illumination slit lamp image depicting central healing anterior stromal infiltrate in a patient with Exserohilum keratitis

10.13.11 Fusarium Solani Keratitis

Fusarium solani keratitis is a severe fungal infection of the cornea caused by *Fusarium solani*. It often presents with symptoms such as pain, redness, and decreased vision. This condition requires prompt antifungal treatment and, in severe cases, surgical intervention to prevent corneal perforation and preserve vision [7].

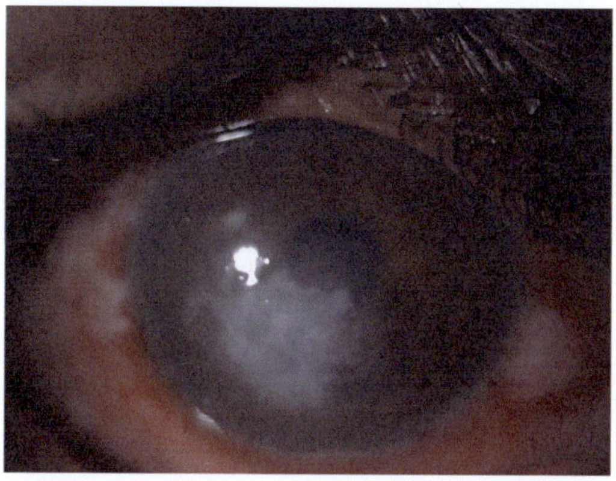

Diffuse illumination slit lamp image depicting anterior stromal infiltrate in a patient with Fusarium solani keratitis

10.13.12 Acanthamoeba Keratitis

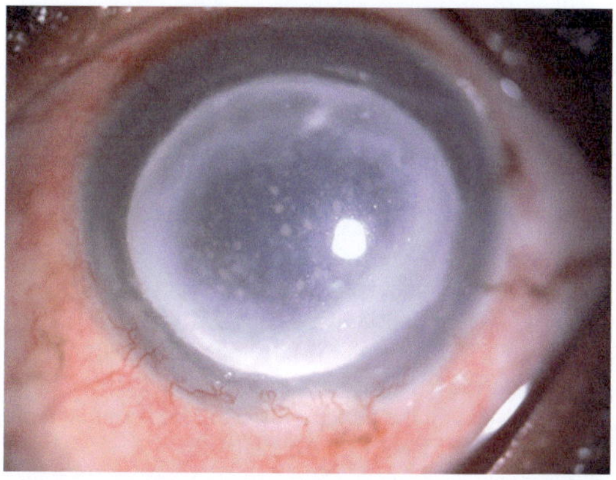

Diffuse illumination slit lamp image depicting ring-shaped near-total corneal infiltrate with keratic precipitates at the back of cornea with superficial corneal vascularization in a patient with Acanthamoeba keratitis

10.13.13 Contact Lens-Induced Keratitis

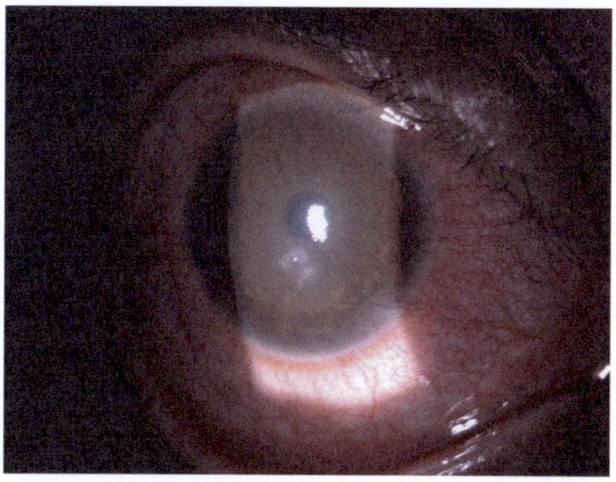

Slit lamp image depicting paracentral anterior stromal infiltrate in a patient with regular contact lens wear

10.13.14 *Candida albicans* Keratitis

Candida albicans keratitis is a fungal infection of the cornea caused by *Candida albicans*. It presents with symptoms such as pain, redness, and decreased vision. Management includes antifungal therapy, and in severe cases, surgical intervention may be necessary to eradicate the infection and restore corneal integrity [32].

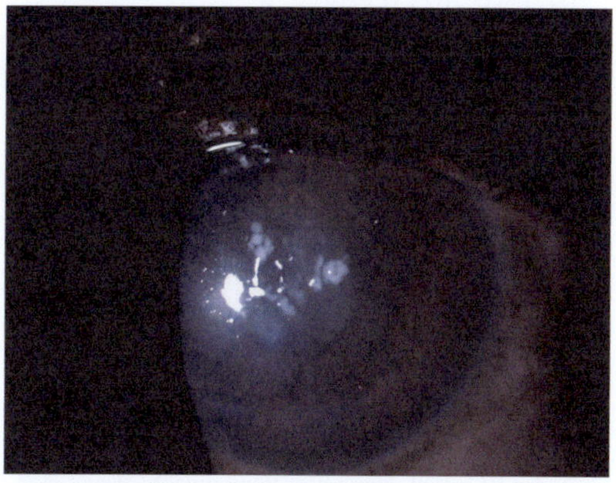

Slit lamp image depicting cheesy anterior stromal infiltrate in a patient affected with *Candida albicans* keratitis

References

1. American Academy of Ophthalmology. Bacterial keratitis preferred practice pattern. San Francisco: American Academy of Ophthalmology; 2018.
2. Green M, Apel A. Infective keratitis. In: Krachmer JH, Mannis MJ, Holland EJ, editors. Cornea. Amsterdam: Elsevier; 2011.
3. Thomas PA, Kaliamurthy J. Mycotic keratitis: epidemiology, diagnosis and management. Clin Microbiol Infect. 2013;19(3):210–20.
4. Gopinathan U, et al. Epidemiological features and laboratory results of fungal keratitis: a 10-year review at a referral eye care center in South India. Cornea. 2002;21(6):555–9.
5. Thomas PA, Kaliamurthy J. Mycotic keratitis: epidemiology, diagnosis, and management. Clin Microbiol Rev. 2013;26(3):557–78.
6. Sridhar MS, et al. Pigmented corneal ulcer caused by Curvularia lunata. Cornea. 2001;20(5):563–5.
7. Gopinathan U, Garg P, Fernandes M, Sharma S, Athmanathan S, Rao GN. The epidemiological features and laboratory results of fungal keratitis: a 10-year review at a referral eye care center in South India. Cornea. 2002;21(6):555–9.
8. Bacon AS, et al. Acanthamoeba keratitis. Ophthalmology. 1993;100(3):403–10.
9. Radford CF, et al. Risk factors for acanthamoeba keratitis in contact lens users: a case-control study. BMJ. 1995;310(6994):1567–70.
10. Gurnani B, Christy J, Kaur K, Moutappa F, Gubert J. Successful management of *Pythium insidiosum* keratitis masquerading as dematiaceous fungal keratitis in an immunosuppressed asian male. Ocul Immunol Inflamm. 2024;32(5):583–6. https://doi.org/10.1080/09273948.2023.2179495.
11. Gurnani B, Natarajan R, Mohan M, Kaur K. Breaking-down barriers: proposal of using cellulose biosynthesis inhibitors and cellulase enzyme as a novel treatment modality for vision threatening pythium insidiosum keratitis. Clin Ophthalmol. 2024;18:765–76. https://doi.org/10.2147/OPTH.S450665. PMID: 38495678; PMCID: PMC10941664.
12. Schein OD, et al. The relative risk of ulcerative keratitis among users of daily-wear and extended-wear soft contact lenses. N Engl J Med. 1989;321(12):773–8.
13. Jacobs DJ, et al. Nontuberculous mycobacterial keratitis: outcomes and treatment. Am J Ophthalmol. 2006;142(6):954–7.
14. Fader RC, et al. Nontuberculous mycobacterial keratitis: diagnosis and management. Ophthalmology. 1990;97(1):130–4.
15. Das S, et al. Microsporidial keratoconjunctivitis in patients with HIV infection in India. J Infect. 2010;61(2):167–8.
16. Gangopadhyay N, et al. Postoperative infections in manual small incision cataract surgery. Indian J Ophthalmol. 2009;57(1):45–9.
17. Price MO, et al. Graft infections after penetrating keratoplasty. Cornea. 2003;22(1):10–3.
18. Watson SL, et al. Peripheral ulcerative keratitis and graft infections after penetrating keratoplasty. Cornea. 2006;25(4):396–9.
19. Sainz de la Maza M, Foster CS, Jabbur NS, Sainz M, Morgan KS. Ocular characteristics and disease associations in the diagnosis of peripheral ulcerative keratitis. Arch Ophthalmol. 2002;120(8):1031–8.
20. Srinivasan M, et al. Ocular morbidity due to late diagnosis of infectious keratitis post-manual small incision cataract surgery. Eye. 2005;19(3):269–74.
21. Pandrowala H, et al. Descemetocele formation in infectious keratitis. Br J Ophthalmol. 2001;85(9):1176–80.
22. Lalitha P, et al. Nocardia keratitis: species, drug sensitivities, and clinical correlation. Cornea. 2003;22(6):476–9.
23. El-Sayed MS, et al. Curvularia keratitis: a case series. Cornea. 2005;24(7):853–5.
24. Austin A, Lietman T. Corneal scraping in the management of infectious keratitis. J Cataract Refract Surg. 2004;30(6):1126–7.
25. Wilhelmus KR. Review of clinical experience with microbial keratitis associated with crystalline keratopathy. Cornea. 2004;23(5):447–9.
26. Dua HS, King AJ, Joseph A. A new classification of ocular surface burns. Br J Ophthalmol. 2001;85(11):1379–83.
27. Wagoner MD, Kenyon KR, Hetherington J. Adhesive use in the treatment of corneal perforations and ulcers. Ophthalmology. 1989;96(5):585–93.
28. O'Brien TP, Maguire MG, Fink NE, Alfonso E, McDonnell P. Efficacy of ofloxacin vs cefazolin and tobramycin in the therapy for bacterial keratitis. Arch Ophthalmol. 1995;113(10):1257–65.
29. Gurnani B, Kaur K, Venugopal A, et al. Pythium insidiosum keratitis - a review. Indian J Ophthalmol. 2022;70(4):1107–20.
30. Hyndiuk RA, Eiferman RA, Caldwell DR, Rosenwasser GO, Gomes JA, Caldwell VR, et al. Comparison of ciprofloxacin ophthalmic solution 0.3% and fortified tobramycin-cefazolin in treating bacterial corneal ulcers. Ciprofloxacin Bacterial Keratitis Study Group. Ophthalmology. 1996;103(11):1854–62.
31. Garg P, Vemuganti GK, Gopinathan U, Naduvilath TJ, Rao GN. Keratomycosis: clinical and microbiologic experience with dematiaceous fungi. Ophthalmology. 2000;107(3):574–80.
32. Thomas PA, Leck AK, Myatt M. Characteristic clinical features as an aid to the diagnosis of suppurative keratitis caused by filamentous fungi. Br J Ophthalmol. 2005;89(12):1554–8.

11 Diagnosis and Management of Immune-Related Disorders of the Cornea and External Eye

Aditi Parab and Josephine Christy S.

11.1 Introduction

Immune-related disorders of the cornea and external eye encompass a diverse group of conditions characterized by inflammatory and immune-mediated processes. These disorders can lead to significant ocular morbidity and vision loss if not appropriately managed. This introduction outlines the clinical features, diagnostic approaches, and management strategies for various immune-related ocular conditions, including peripheral ulcerative keratitis, Mooren's ulcer, blepharitis, marginal keratitis, Stevens-Johnson syndrome, episcleritis, scleritis, Thygeson's superficial punctate keratitis, interstitial keratitis, ligneous conjunctivitis, contact dermatoblepharitis, allergic conjunctivitis, vernal keratoconjunctivitis, and scleritis.

11.2 Peripheral Ulcerative Keratitis

11.2.1 Crescentic Guttering

Peripheral ulcerative keratitis (PUK) is an inflammatory condition of the peripheral cornea associated with systemic autoimmune diseases such as rheumatoid arthritis and systemic lupus erythematosus. Clinically, PUK presents with peripheral corneal thinning, ulceration, and an overlying epithelial defect. Diagnosis involves clinical examination, systemic evaluation, and laboratory tests to identify underlying systemic diseases. Management includes local and systemic immunosuppressive therapy, along with antimicrobial prophylaxis to prevent secondary infections [1, 2].

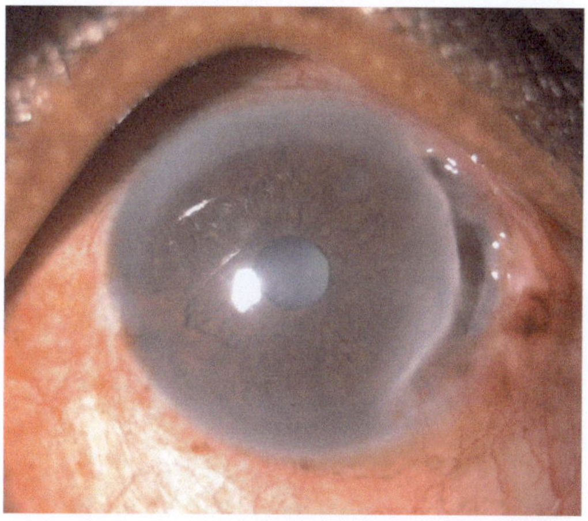

Figure illustrating crescent-shaped destructive thinning of juxtalimbal corneal stroma classical of peripheral ulcerative keratitis

A. Parab · J. Christy S. (✉)
Cornea and Refractive Services, Aravind Eye Hospital and Post Graduate Institute of Ophthalmology, Pondicherry, India

B. Gurnani, K. Kaur (eds.), *Atlas of Cornea*, https://doi.org/10.1007/978-981-96-0013-7_11

11.2.2 Guttering with Infiltration

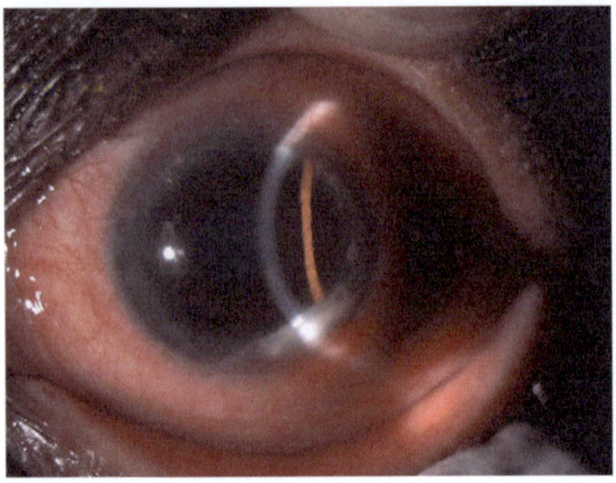

Figure illustrating inferonasal crescent-shaped destructive thinning of anterior corneal stroma suggestive of peripheral ulcerative keratitis

11.2.3 Mooren's Ulcer

Mooren's ulcer is a rare, idiopathic, peripheral corneal ulceration with an autoimmune etiology. It presents with progressive, painful peripheral corneal ulceration without scleritis. Diagnosis is clinical, supported by the exclusion of other causes of peripheral ulceration. Treatment includes topical and systemic immunosuppressive agents and surgical interventions such as conjunctival resection or amniotic membrane transplantation in refractory cases [3, 4].

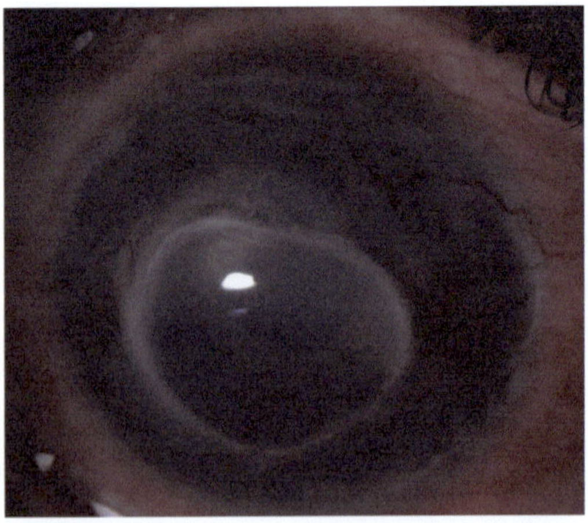

Figure showing Mooren's ulcer characterized by peripheral corneal thinning which progresses first circumferentially and then centrally; vascularization is seen at the bed of the furrow

11.2.4 Blepharitis

Blepharitis is a common inflammatory condition affecting the eyelids, characterized by chronic irritation, redness, and crusting at the eyelid margins. It can be anterior (affecting the base of the eyelashes) or posterior (affecting the meibomian glands). Diagnosis is clinical, and management includes eyelid hygiene, topical antibiotics, and anti-inflammatory agents [5].

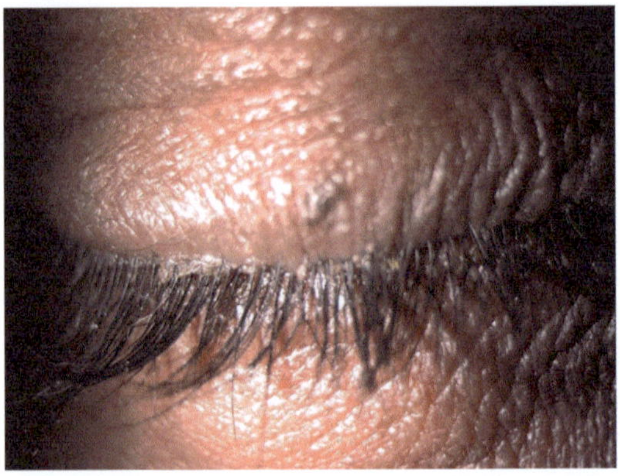

Figure illustrating dandruff-like flakes or crusts at the base of the eyelashes causing inflammation of the eyelids called as blepharitis

11.2.5 Marginal Keratitis

Marginal keratitis is an inflammatory condition often associated with chronic blepharitis. It presents as peripheral corneal infiltrates adjacent to the limbus with overlying epithelial defects. Diagnosis is based on clinical findings and exclusion of infectious causes. Treatment includes managing the underlying blepharitis and using topical corticosteroids to reduce inflammation [6].

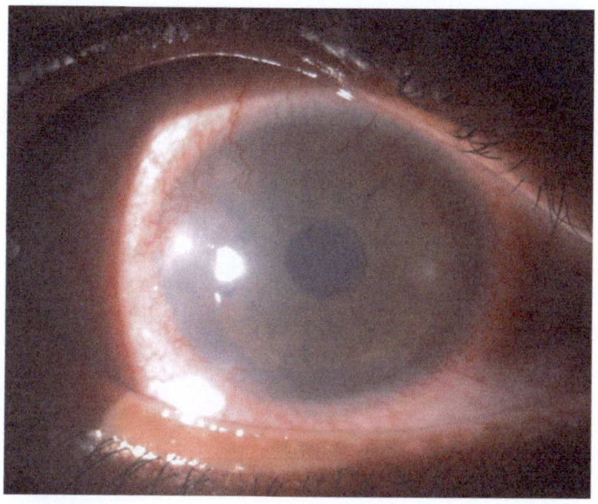

Figure illustrating marginal keratitis characterized by peripheral stromal infiltrate with superficial vascularization indicating chronicity of the condition

11.2.6 Stevens-Johnson Syndrome

Stevens-Johnson syndrome (SJS) is a severe mucocutaneous disorder often triggered by medications or infections. Ocular involvement includes conjunctivitis, keratitis, and corneal ulceration. Diagnosis is clinical, with support from histopathological findings. Management involves supportive care, discontinuation of the offending agent, and ocular surface protection using lubricants, topical steroids, and, in severe cases, surgical interventions like amniotic membrane transplantation [7, 8].

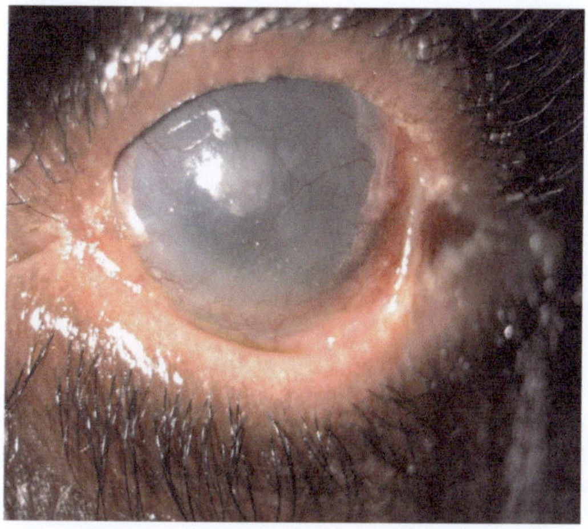

Figure illustrating ocular SJS manifesting as limbal stem cell deficiency with corneal opacification, dry ocular surface, lid margin keratinization, and symblepharon formation

11.2.7 Episcleritis

Episcleritis is a benign, self-limiting inflammation of the episclera, presenting with sectoral redness and mild discomfort. In contrast, scleritis is a severe, potentially vision-threatening inflammation of the sclera, associated with systemic autoimmune diseases. Diagnosis is clinical, supported by imaging and laboratory tests to identify underlying systemic conditions. Management includes topical or systemic anti-inflammatory agents for episcleritis and systemic immunosuppressive therapy for scleritis [9, 10].

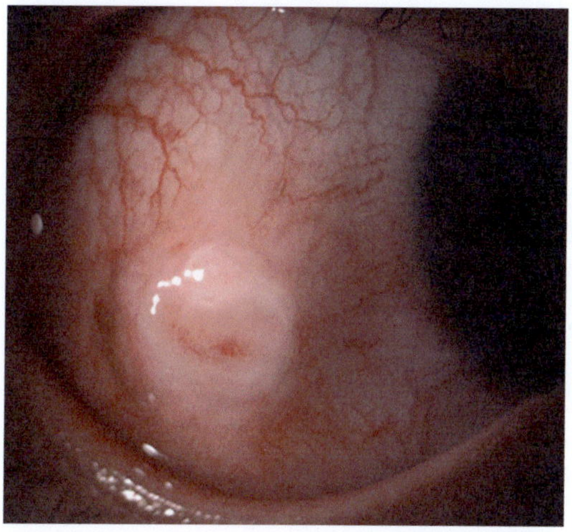

Figure showing nodular episcleritis characterized by dilated and congested episcleral vessels with a nodular discrete elevated area of episcleral tissue

11.2.8 Scleritis

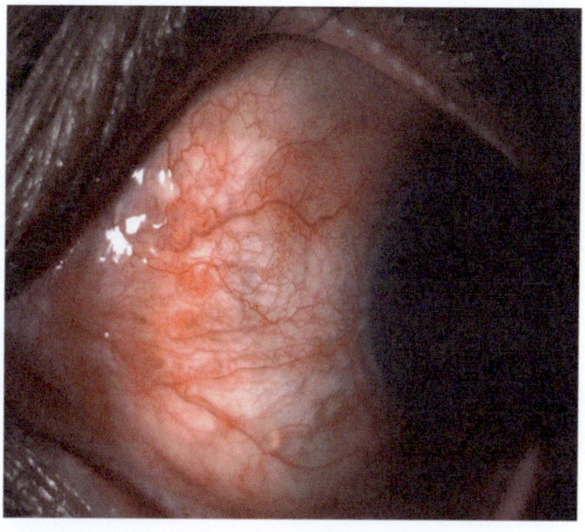

Figure illustrating anterior scleritis characterized by anterior scleral edema with dilatation of deep episcleral vessels

11.2.9 Thygeson's Superficial Punctate Keratitis

Thygeson's superficial punctate keratitis is a chronic, recurrent condition characterized by multiple, small, epithelial lesions on the cornea. Diagnosis is clinical, and treatment includes lubricants and topical corticosteroids to reduce inflammation during acute episodes [11].

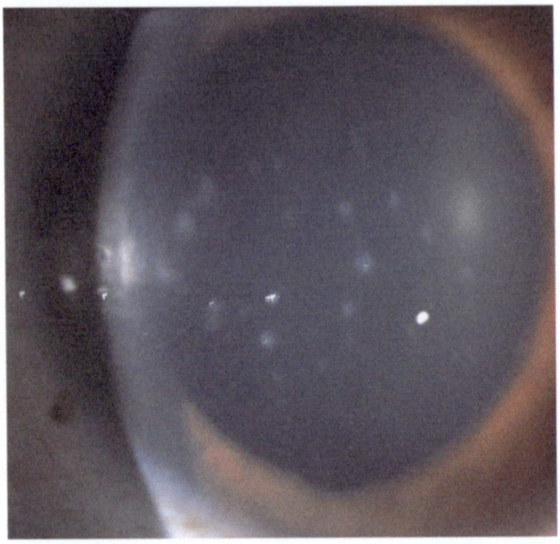

Figure showing multiple small and elevated intraepithelial grayish white opacities, classical of Thygeson's superficial punctate keratitis

11.2.10 Interstitial Keratitis

Interstitial keratitis is an inflammation of the corneal stroma without primary involvement of the epithelium or endothelium, often associated with systemic infections like syphilis. Diagnosis includes clinical examination, serological tests, and imaging studies. Management involves treating the underlying infection and using anti-inflammatory agents to control stromal inflammation [12].

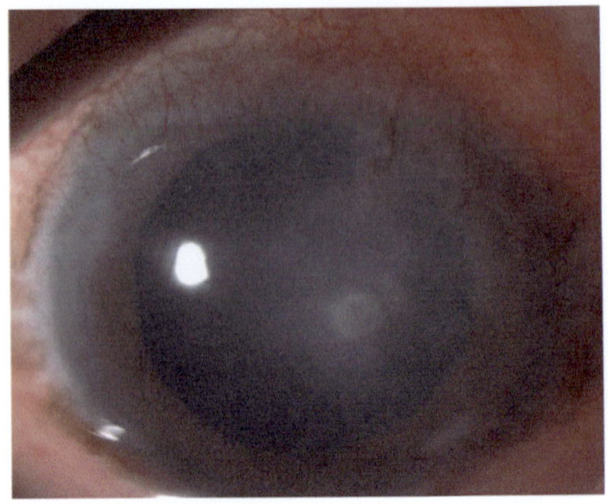

Figure showing stromal haze with infiltrate and neovascularization of the cornea, commonly seen as late sequelae of congenital or acquired syphilis

11.2.11 Ligneous Conjunctivitis

Ligneous conjunctivitis is a rare, chronic condition characterized by wood-like pseudomembranes on the conjunctiva, often associated with plasminogen deficiency. Diagnosis is based on clinical features and laboratory tests for plasminogen levels. Treatment includes surgical removal of the pseudomembranes and topical plasminogen replacement therapy [13].

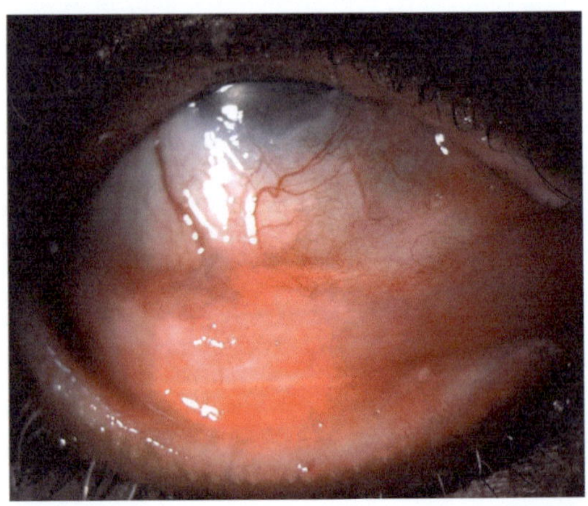

Figure illustrating fibrinous pseudomembranes on the lower palpebral conjunctiva, a typical finding of ligneous conjunctivitis

11.2.12 Contact Dermatoblepharitis

Contact dermatoblepharitis and allergic conjunctivitis are inflammatory conditions resulting from hypersensitivity reactions to allergens. Symptoms include itching, redness, and swelling of the eyelids and conjunctiva. Diagnosis is clinical, supported by allergy testing. Management involves avoiding the allergen, using topical antihistamines, and corticosteroids for severe cases [14, 15].

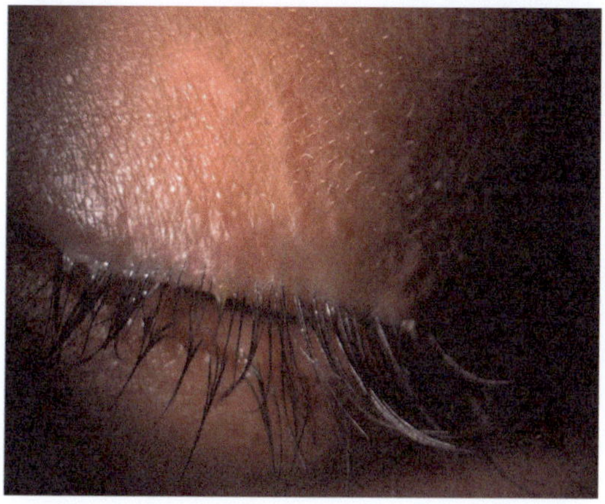

Figure showing matted eyelashes with erythematous, thickened, and scaly skin following contact with topical ophthalmic medication

11.2.13 Allergic Conjunctivitis

Allergic conjunctivitis is an inflammation of the conjunctiva caused by allergic reactions to environmental allergens such as pollen, dust mites, or animal dander. Symptoms include itching, redness, tearing, and swelling. Management includes avoiding allergens and using antihistamines or anti-inflammatory medications to relieve symptoms [16].

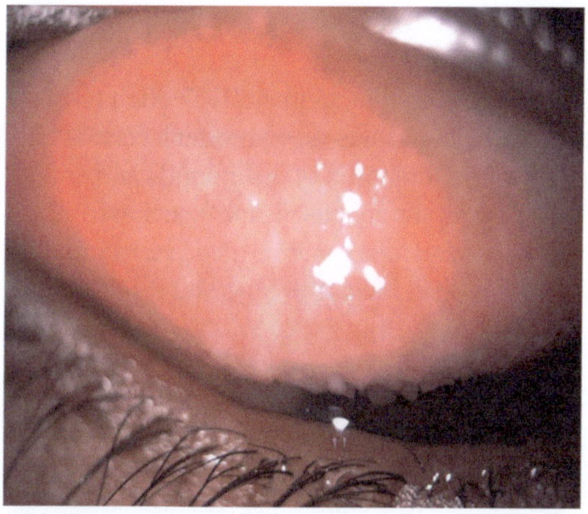

Figure showing papillae in upper tarsal conjunctiva with edematous and hyperemic conjunctiva, seen in allergic conjunctivitis

11.3 Vernal Keratoconjunctivitis

11.3.1 Giant Papillae

Vernal keratoconjunctivitis (VKC) is a chronic, seasonal allergic condition affecting young individuals. It presents with severe itching, photophobia, and large papillae on the tarsal conjunctiva. Diagnosis is clinical, and treatment includes mast cell stabilizers, antihistamines, and topical corticosteroids for acute exacerbations [17].

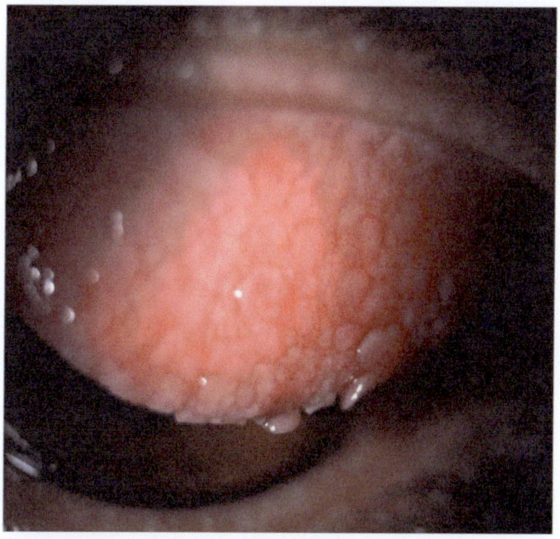

Figure showing discrete >1 mm diameter flat-topped giant papillae in a case of vernal keratoconjunctivitis

11.3.2 Horner-Trantas Spots

Vernal keratoconjunctivitis (VKC) often presents with Horner-Trantas spots, which are white, chalky dots composed of eosinophils and epithelial debris at the limbus. These spots are indicative of severe inflammation and are commonly associated with intense itching and discomfort in VKC patients [18].

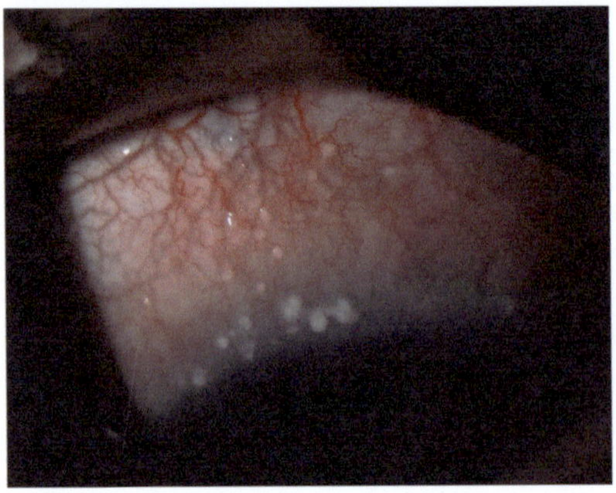

Figure showing whitish dots in the perilimbal region consisting of degenerated epithelial cells and eosinophils

11.3.3 Limbal Papillae

Vernal keratoconjunctivitis (VKC) frequently involves the development of limbal papillae, which are elevated, gelatinous nodules at the limbus. These papillae are a result of chronic allergic inflammation and can cause significant discomfort, photophobia, and visual impairment if left untreated [18].

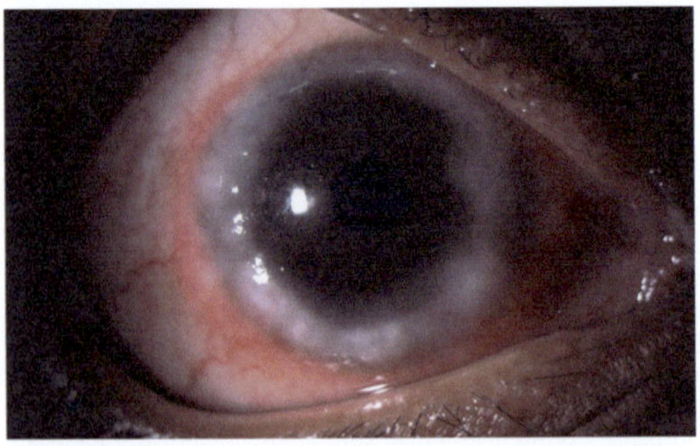

Figure showing limbal hyperplasia with limbal papillae which are the accumulation of lymphocytes at the limbus

11.3.4 Shield Ulcer

Vernal keratoconjunctivitis (VKC) can lead to the formation of shield ulcers, which are large, superficial corneal epithelial defects. These ulcers result from chronic inflammation and mechanical trauma due to eye rubbing, requiring treatment with anti-inflammatory medications and therapeutic contact lenses to promote healing and prevent scarring [18].

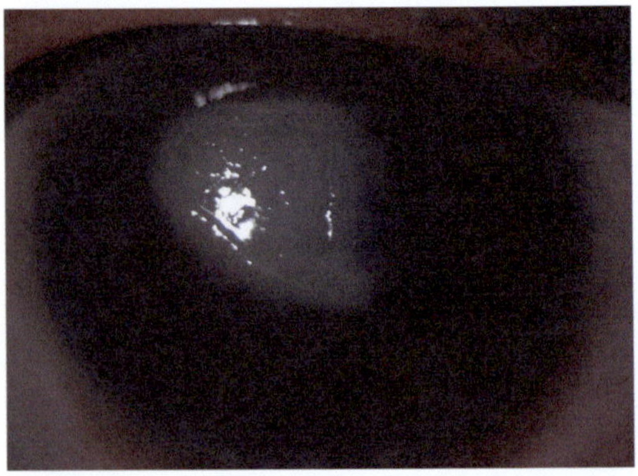

Figure illustrating shield ulcer which is a macro-erosion with the deposition of plaque containing fibrin and mucus

11.3.5 Scleral Melt in Scleritis

Scleral melt in scleritis is a severe complication characterized by the progressive thinning and necrosis of the scleral tissue, often leading to perforation. This condition requires aggressive immunosuppressive therapy to control the underlying inflammation and prevent further tissue destruction [1].

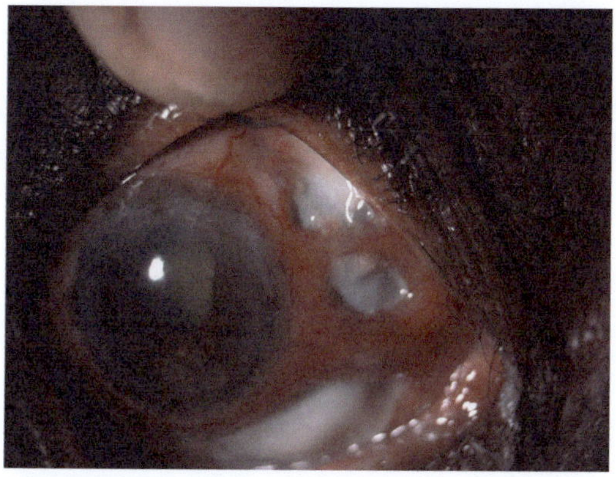

Diffuse illumination slit lamp image of a patient depicting pus-filled scleral pockets with melt along with scleral inflammation

11.3.6 Scleral Abscess with Scleritis

A scleral abscess with scleritis is a severe infection characterized by localized pus formation within the sclera accompanied by intense inflammation. This condition can lead to significant pain, redness, and potential vision loss, requiring urgent antimicrobial therapy and possibly surgical drainage to control the infection and prevent further complications [19].

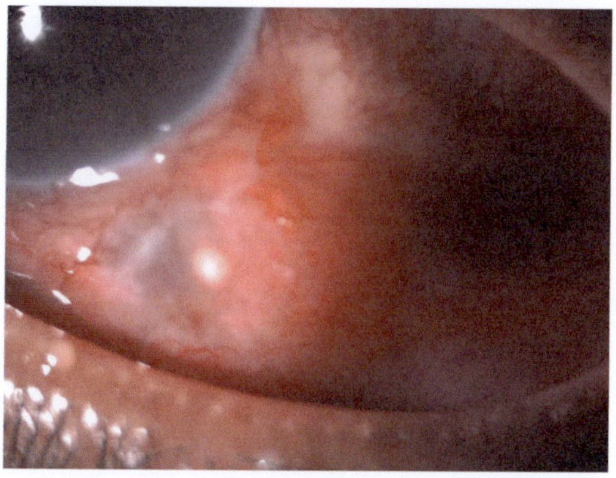

Diffuse illumination slit lamp image of a patient depicting pus-filled scleral pockets with melt along with scleritis

11.3.7 Corneal Neovascularization in Dry Eyes

Corneal neovascularization in dry eyes occurs due to chronic inflammation and hypoxia, leading to the growth of new blood vessels into the cornea. This condition can cause visual impairment and discomfort, requiring treatments such as anti-inflammatory medications, lubricants, and, in severe cases, anti-VEGF therapy to inhibit neovascularization [20].

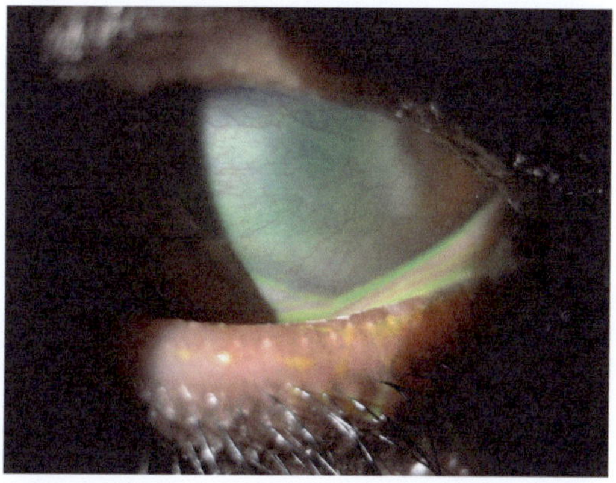

Diffuse illumination slit lamp image of a patient depicting superficial and deep corneal vascularization along with corneal scar in a patient with dry eyes

References

1. Watson PG, Hayreh SS. Scleritis and episcleritis. Br J Ophthalmol. 1976;60(3):163–91.
2. Foster CS. Immunosuppressive therapy for external ocular inflammatory disease. Ophthalmology. 1980;87(2):140–50.
3. Ladas JG, Mondino BJ. Systemic disorders associated with peripheral corneal ulceration. Curr Opin Ophthalmol. 2000;11(6):468–71.
4. Srinivasan M, Zegans ME, Kundu A, et al. Clinical characteristics of Mooren's ulcer in South India. Br J Ophthalmol. 2007;91(5):570–5.
5. Lemp MA, Nichols KK. Blepharitis in the United States 2009: a survey-based perspective on prevalence and treatment. Ocul Surf. 2009;7(2):S1–S14.
6. Wong AH, et al. Marginal keratitis and its association with blepharitis. Eye Contact Lens. 2014;40(5):335–8.

7. Chang YS, et al. Stevens-Johnson syndrome and toxic epidermal necrolysis in children. J Dermatol. 2016;43(5):512–7.
8. Sotozono C, et al. Management of Stevens-Johnson syndrome and toxic epidermal necrolysis with ocular complications. Ophthalmology. 2009;116(4):685–90.
9. Watson PG. Episcleritis and scleritis. Trans Ophthalmol Soc Aust. 1973;93(4):579–96.
10. Akpek EK, et al. Evaluation of patients with scleritis for systemic disease. Ophthalmology. 2004;111(3):501–6.
11. Thygeson P. Superficial punctate keratitis. JAMA J Am Med Assoc. 1950;144(18):1544–9.
12. Dana MR, et al. Interstitial keratitis and recurrent corneal erosion associated with Epstein-Barr virus. Cornea. 1996;15(5):537–42.
13. Schuster V, et al. Plasminogen deficiency. J Thromb Haemost. 2007;5(12):2315–22.
14. Bielory L. Allergic conjunctivitis: the evolution of therapeutic options. Allergy Asthma Proc. 2012;33(2):129–39.
15. Abelson MB, et al. Allergic conjunctivitis. Surv Ophthalmol. 1980;24(6):367–76.
16. Bielory L. Allergic conjunctivitis: the evolution of therapy and challenges ahead. Curr Allergy Asthma Rep. 2010;10(2):105–14.
17. Leonardi A, et al. Vernal keratoconjunctivitis: pathogenesis and treatment. Prog Retin Eye Res. 2004;23(3):195–228.
18. Bonini S, Coassin M, Aronni S, Lambiase A. Vernal keratoconjunctivitis. Eye. 2004;18(4):345–51.
19. Espana EM, Foster CS. Scleral infections. Int Ophthalmol Clin. 2003;43(2):149–65.
20. Jeng BH, Dupps WJ. Autologous serum 50% eye drops in the treatment of persistent corneal epithelial defects and ulcers. Cornea. 2009;28(10):1104–8.

12 Neoplastic Disorders of the Conjunctiva and Cornea

Rolika Bansal and Santosh G. Honavar

12.1 Introduction

Neoplastic disorders of the conjunctiva and cornea encompass a spectrum of benign and malignant growths that can significantly impact ocular health and vision. These conditions range from relatively innocuous lesions to aggressive malignancies requiring prompt and accurate management. This introduction covers various neoplastic disorders, including conjunctival papilloma, conjunctival nevus, pyogenic granuloma, limbal dermoid, dermolipoma, ocular surface squamous neoplasia (OSSN), sebaceous gland carcinoma, nevus of Ota, and malignant melanoma.

12.2 Conjunctival Papilloma

Conjunctival papillomas are benign epithelial tumors often associated with human papilloma virus (HPV) infection. They present as sessile or pedunculated lesions on the conjunctiva, commonly near the limbus or fornices. Diagnosis is typically clinical, supplemented by histopathological confirmation. Management involves surgical excision, with adjuvant cryotherapy or topical antivirals for recurrent cases [1, 2].

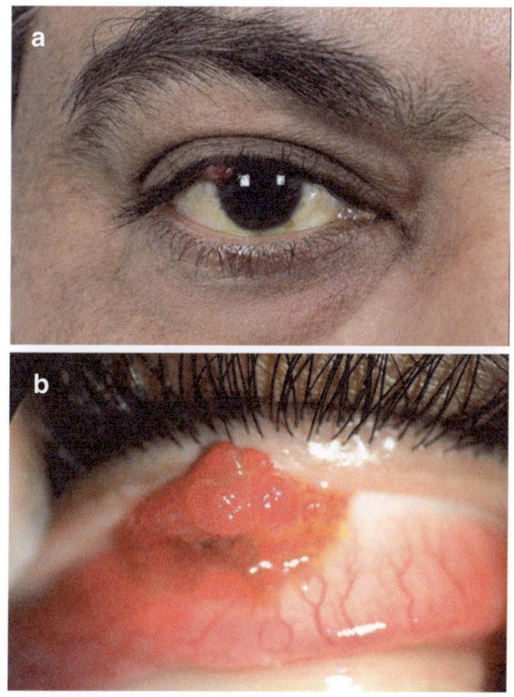

(**a**) A 42-year-old male presented with a right upper eyelid vascular lesion at the junction of medial two-third and lateral one-third. (**b**) On the upper eyelid eversion, the lesion appeared vascular and sessile with a corrugated surface, confirming the diagnosis as a conjunctival papilloma

R. Bansal · S. G. Honavar (✉)
CFS Education, CFS Hyderabad,
Hyderabad, Andhra Pradesh, India

B. Gurnani, K. Kaur (eds.), *Atlas of Cornea*, https://doi.org/10.1007/978-981-96-0013-7_12

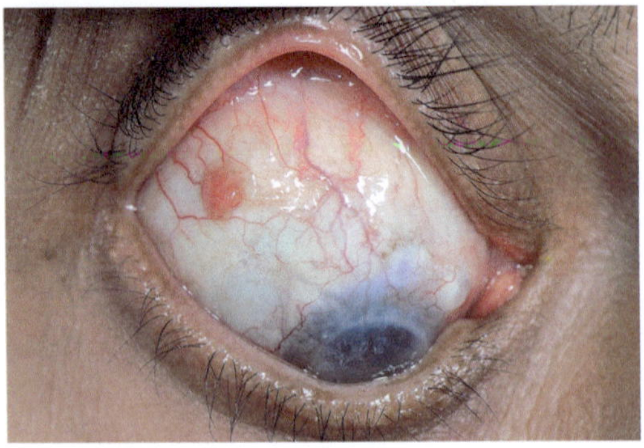

A 72-year-old female presented with a tiny conjunctival sessile papilloma in the superotemporal bulbar region

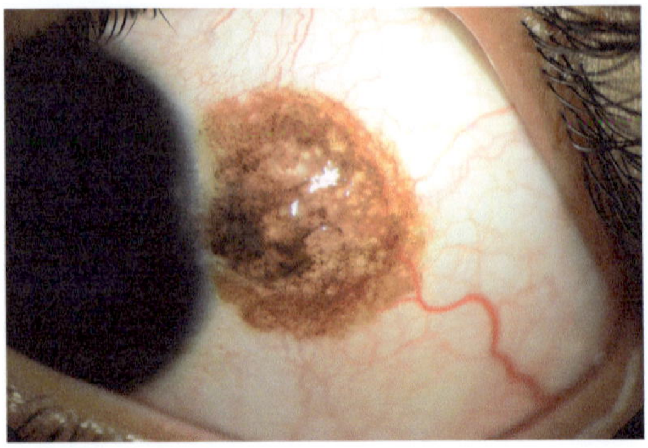

A 25-year-old female presented with a pigmented lesion in the temporal bulbar perilimbal region with variable pigmentation and cystic changes with a prominent feeder vessel. The variable pigmentation indicates toward the diagnosis of a conjunctival nevus

12.3 Conjunctival Nevus

A conjunctival nevus is a common benign melanocytic lesion appearing during childhood or adolescence. These nevi are usually pigmented and can occur anywhere on the conjunctiva, frequently near the limbus. While generally asymptomatic, they require regular monitoring for any signs of malignant transformation. While observation is preferred, in cases with suspected growth or malignancy, excision biopsy is performed with histopathological confirmation [3, 4].

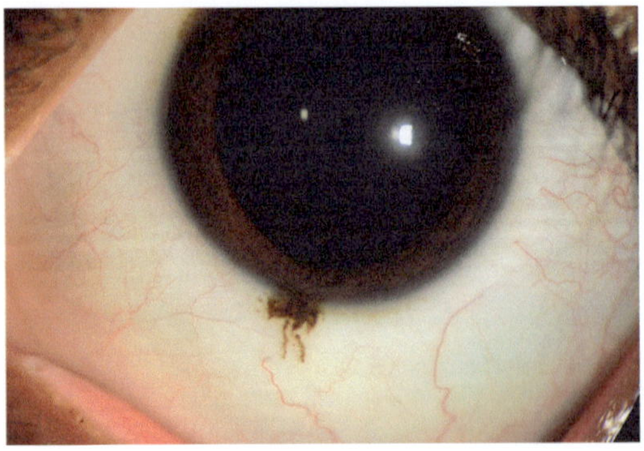

A 15-year-old male presented with a pigmented lesion in the perilimbal region with variable pigmentation, thus indicating a diagnosis of a conjunctival nevus

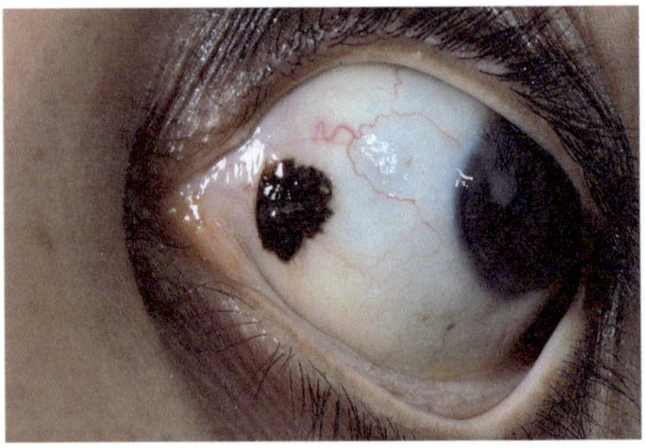

A 15-year-old male presented with a dark, deeply pigmented lesion in the nasal bulbar region with cystic spaces which was treated with excision biopsy, and the histopathology confirmed the diagnosis of conjunctival nevus

12.4 Pyogenic Granuloma

Pyogenic granuloma is a reactive, vascular lesion often arising after trauma, surgery, or inflammation. It presents as a rapidly growing, red, fleshy mass on the conjunctiva. Although benign, it can cause discomfort and bleeding. Diagnosis is clinical, and treatment involves topical steroids to reduce inflammation and surgical excision for residual lesions [5].

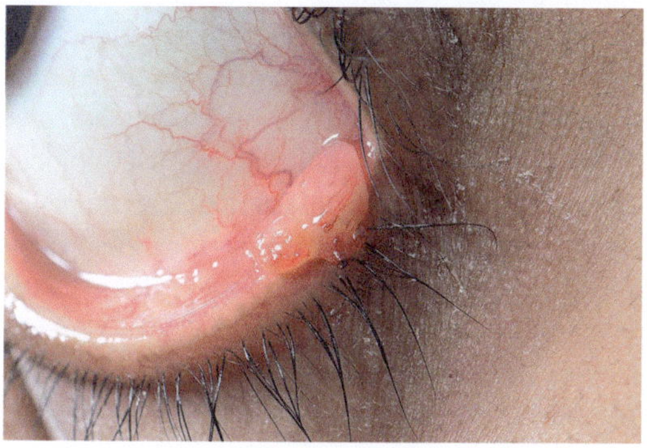

A 34-year-old male presented with a vascular pedunculated lesion with a tendency to bleed on touch in the inferior fornix of the left eye. These features indicate toward the diagnosis of pyogenic granuloma

12.4.1 Limbal Dermoid

Limbal dermoids and dermolipomas are congenital choristomas, presenting as benign, well-circumscribed masses containing tissues such as hair, fat, and cartilage. Limbal dermoids typically occur at the corneoscleral junction, while dermolipomas are found in the superotemporal quadrant. These lesions can cause visual impairment and cosmetic concerns. Surgical excision is the treatment of choice, particularly if the lesion interferes with vision or causes significant discomfort [6, 7].

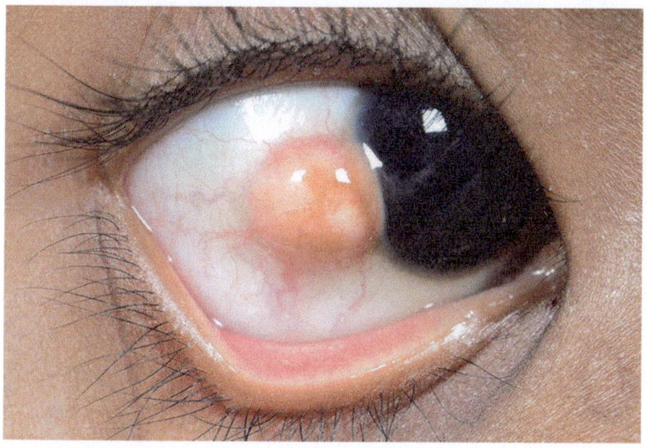

A 17-year-old female presented with a perilimbal lesion in the inferotemporal quadrant with a corneal overlap. This is highly suggestive of a limbal dermoid

12.4.2 Dermolipoma

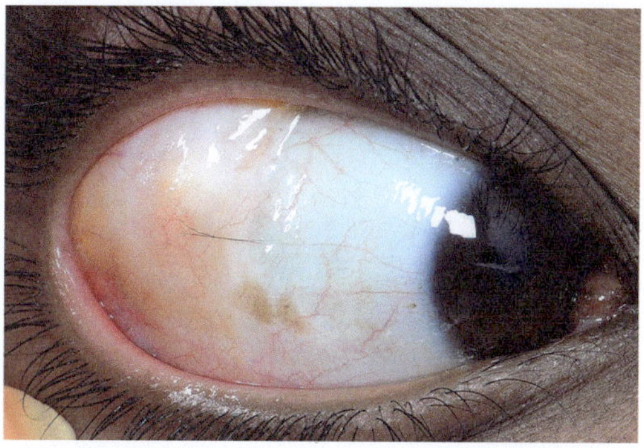

A 32-year-old male presented with a superotemporal forniceal bulge with overlying hair shafts and yellowish hue indicating underlying fatty components. This is suggestive of a dermolipoma

12.5 Ocular Surface Squamous Neoplasia

Ocular Surface Squamous Neoplasia (OSSN) of the cornea and conjunctiva is a malignant tumor characterized by the abnormal growth of squamous cells. It often presents as a raised, gelatinous lesion on the ocular surface and can lead to significant morbidity if not treated promptly.

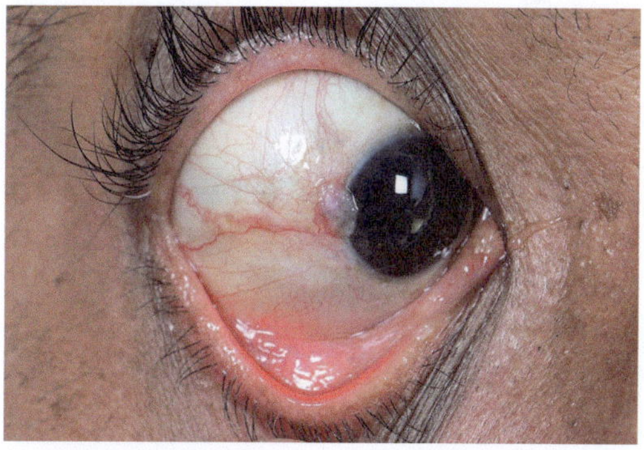

A 49-year-old male presented with a pinkish lesion in the temporal perilimbal region with overlying leukoplakia and a prominent feeder vessel, thus indicating ocular surface squamous neoplasia

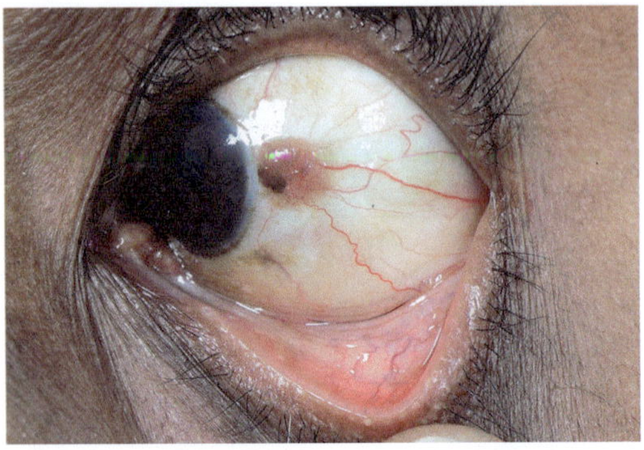

A 52-year-old male presented with a pinkish lesion with an overlying pigmented component in the temporal perilimbal region of the left eye with a prominent feeder vessel, thus indicating ocular surface squamous neoplasia

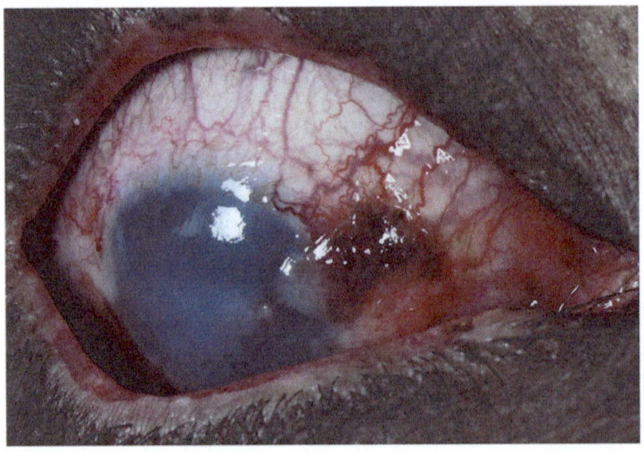

A 14-year-old male with xeroderma pigmentosa presented with a diffuse vascular conjunctival lesion with a cornea overlap and prominent feeder vessels. This suggests a diffuse ocular surface squamous neoplasia with corneal overlap

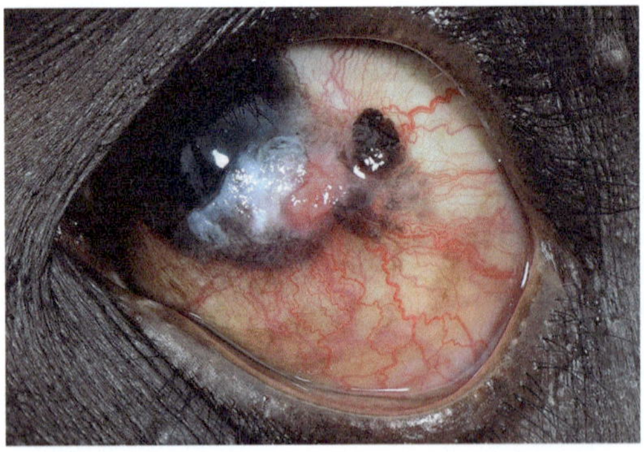

A 45-year-old male presented with a conjunctival vascular lesion, pigmented component, corneal overlap, leukoplakia, and dilated feeder vessels, which was treated with excision biopsy with keratectomy with 4 mm clinically clear margins, and the histopathology confirmed the diagnosis of ocular surface squamous neoplasia

OSSN encompasses a range of dysplastic and neoplastic epithelial lesions, including conjunctival intraepithelial neoplasia (CIN) and invasive squamous cell carcinoma. Risk factors include UV exposure, HPV infection, and immunosuppression. Clinically, OSSN presents as an elevated, gelatinous lesion on the ocular surface. Diagnosis is confirmed through histopathological analysis. Treatment includes medical management with topical chemotherapy or surgical excision with no-touch technique along with cryotherapy. In cases with corneal involvement, alcohol keratoepitheliectomy should be performed. In extensive cases immunotherapy may be performed [8, 9].

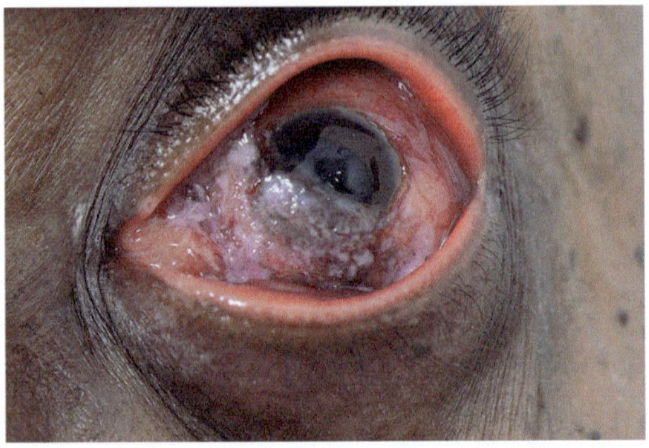

A 54-year-old male shows a more diffuse involvement of ocular surface squamous neoplasia with an orbital component, thus indicating the need for exenteration

12.6 Sebaceous Gland Carcinoma

Sebaceous gland carcinoma is a rare, aggressive malignancy originating from the meibomian glands or glands of Zeis. It often masquerades as benign conditions like chalazia or blepharoconjunctivitis, leading to delayed diagnosis. This carcinoma can present with a yellowish nodular mass, diffuse thickening of the eyelid margin, or chronic unilateral conjunctivitis. Management requires wide local excision with clinically clear margins along with map biopsy to rule out pagetoid spread.with clinically clear margins along with map biopsy to rule out pagetoid spread [10, 11].

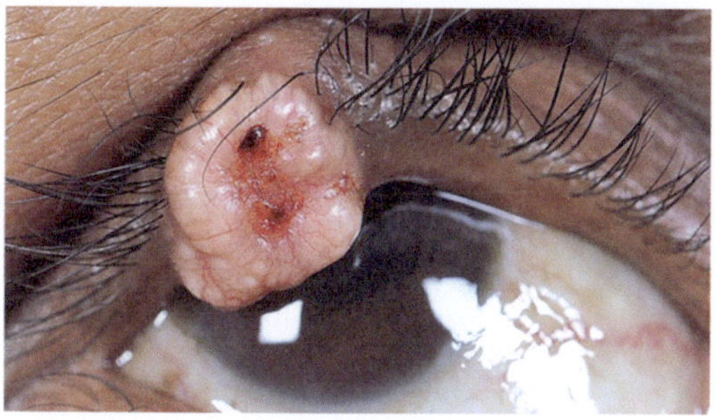

A 51-year-old female shows a right upper eyelid lesion with yellowish nodules, widening of the eyelid margin, and loss of cilia, suggestive of a sebaceous gland carcinoma

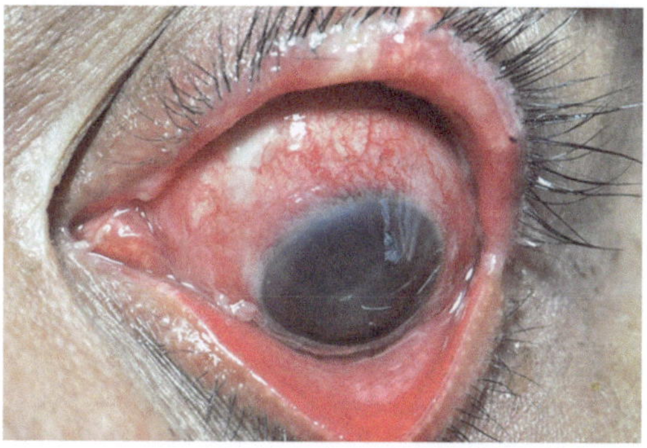

A 63-year-old female presented with a diffuse eyelid and conjunctival involvement with intraepithelial component, suggestive of sebaceous carcinoma with pagetoid spread

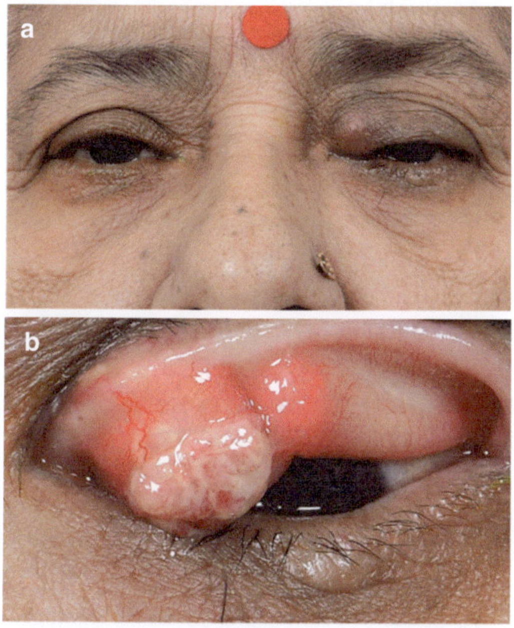

(**a**) A 75-year-old female presented with a nodular lesion in the left upper eyelid extending till the upper tarsal region. (**b**) Left upper eyelid eversion revealed a yellowish nodular crossing the upper edge of the tarsus with intrinsic vascularity and prominent vessels, involving the peripunctal region as well. A final diagnosis of sebaceous carcinoma was made after a wide excision with the reconstruction of the upper eyelid

12.7 Nevus of Ota

Nevus of Ota, or oculodermal melanocytosis, is a congenital hyperpigmentation disorder involving the periocular skin, sclera, and uveal tract. It presents as blue or gray patches, primarily affecting the trigeminal nerve distribution area. Although benign, there is an increased risk of developing melanoma, necessitating regular ophthalmologic examinations [12, 13].

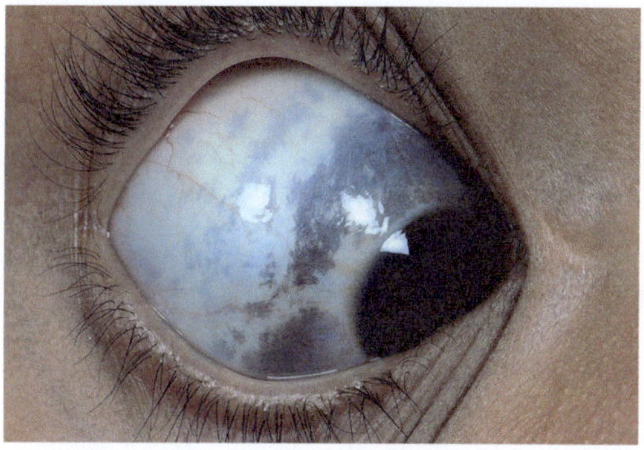

A 9-year-old girl presented with unilateral diffuse conjunctival and scleral pigmentation with 360 degree involvement, suggestive of nevus of Ota

12.8 Malignant Melanoma

Conjunctival malignant melanoma is a rare but highly malignant tumor arising from pre-existing nevi, primary acquired melanosis, or de novo. It presents as a pigmented or nonpigmented nodular lesion, often with feeder vessels. Early diagnosis through clinical examination and imaging is critical. Treatment involves wide local excision with clinically clear margin, adjunctive cryotherapy, and in invasive cases plaque brachytherapy can be performed. Close follow-up with systemic evaluation is essential due to the high risk of recurrence and metastasis [14, 15].

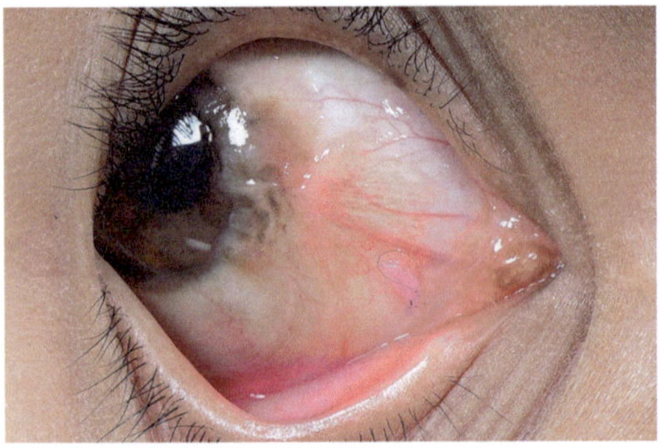

A 42-year-old male presented with a conjunctival lesion with the pigmented component in the perilimbal region which was excised with 4 mm clinically clear margin and confirmed as malignant melanoma on histopathology. Due to the presence of scleral invasion, secondary plaque brachytherapy was performed with excellent outcome

References

1. Shields CL, Shields JA. Tumors of the conjunctiva and cornea. Surv Ophthalmol. 2004;49(1):3–24.
2. Karp CL, Scott IU, Chang TS, Pflugfelder SC. Conjunctival papilloma: clinical features and management. Ophthalmology. 2016;123(3):546–50.
3. Shields JA, Mashayekhi A, Kligman BE, Rudich DS, Marr BP, Shields CL. Conjunctival nevus: clinical features and natural course in 410 consecutive patients. Arch Ophthalmol. 2011;129(8):998–1003.
4. Cockerham KP, Hidayat AA, Jakobiec FA, Zakka FR. Benign conjunctival melanocytic lesions: clinical and pathologic features. Ophthalmology. 2015;122(3):494–9.
5. Granstein RD, Baum CL, Halasz CL. Pyogenic granuloma: its histomorphogenesis and its relationship to other vascular proliferations. J Am Acad Dermatol. 2014;71(5):941–54.
6. Mannis MJ, Brown SI. Congenital dermoid cysts of the limbus. Am J Ophthalmol. 1983;95(5):760–5.
7. Shields JA, Demirci H, Karatza EC, Shields CL. Dermolipoma of the ocular adnexa. Ophthalmic Plast Reconstr Surg. 2013;29(4):261–5.
8. Galor A, Karp CL, Oellers P, Kao AA, Abdelaziz A, Feuer W, et al. Predictors of ocular surface squamous neoplasia recurrence after excisional surgery. Ophthalmology. 2012;119(10):1974–81.
9. Kim HJ, Shields CL, Shah SU, Marr BP, Shields JA. Treatment of ocular surface squamous neoplasia with topical interferon alpha-2b. Ophthalmology. 2012;119(5):938–44.
10. Shields JA, Demirci H, Marr BP, Eagle RC Jr, Shields CL. Sebaceous gland carcinoma of the eyelids: personal experience with 60 cases. Trans Am Ophthalmol Soc. 2005;103:357–68.
11. Shields JA, Demirci H, Marr BP, Eagle RC Jr, Shields CL. Sebaceous gland carcinoma. Review of the literature and classification of 394 cases. Am J Ophthalmol. 2011;150(2):195–204.
12. Teekhasaenee C, Ritch R, Rutnin U, Leelawongs N. Ocular and oculodermal melanocytosis: natural history and malignant transformation. Br J Ophthalmol. 1990;74(11):647–9.
13. Jang HS, Kim YC, Choi HY. Melanocytic nevi and melanoma associated with nevus of Ota. Ann Dermatol. 2015;27(3):366–70.
14. Shields CL, Markowitz JS, Belinsky I, Schwartzstein H, George NS, Lally SE, et al. Conjunctival melanoma: outcomes based on tumor origin in 382 consecutive cases. Ophthalmology. 2011;118(2):389–95.
15. Esmaeli B, Papadopoulos NE, Kim EY, Wang X, Wolf A, Hwu WJ, et al. Conjunctival melanoma: histopathologic features predictive of metastasis and death in 150 patients. Clin Cancer Res. 2015;21(13):3163–9.

Clinical Aspects of Toxic and Traumatic Injuries of the Anterior Segment

13

Anitha Venugopal, Bharat Gurnani, and Kirandeep Kaur

13.1 Introduction

Toxic and traumatic injuries to the anterior segment of the eye encompass a range of conditions that can lead to significant ocular morbidity and vision impairment. The anterior segment, comprising structures such as the cornea, iris, ciliary body, and lens, is particularly vulnerable to various forms of injury. This introduction reviews the clinical aspects of several key conditions, including iridodialysis, corneal perforation, limbal tear, scleral tear, hyphema, corneal abrasions, toxic keratopathy, multiple corneal foreign bodies, superficial corneal foreign body, deep anterior lamellar keratoplasty, post-corneal tear repair with iris abscission, thermal injury, toxic endotheliitis, intralenticular abscess, traumatic cataract, traumatic dislocation of the LASIK flap, pseudophacocele, therapeutic penetrating keratoplasty, and optical penetrating keratoplasty.

13.2 Iridodialysis

13.2.1 Large Dialysis with Hyphema

Iridodialysis is the disinsertion of the iris from its attachment at the ciliary body, typically resulting from blunt trauma. Patients present with monocular diplopia, photophobia, and potential visual field defects. Diagnosis is clinical, confirmed by slit lamp examination revealing the iris disinsertion. Management may involve surgical repair for significant cases or cosmetic contact lenses for minor cases [1, 2].

A. Venugopal (✉)
Cornea, Ocular Surface, Trauma and Refractive, Services, Aravind Eye Hospital and Postgraduate Institute of Ophthalmology, Tirunelveli, Tamil Nadu, India
e-mail: dranitha@aravind.org

B. Gurnani
Department of Cataract, Cornea, Trauma, External Diseases, Ocular Surface and Refractive Services, Gomabai Netralaya and Research Centre, Neemuch, Madhya Pradesh, India

K. Kaur
Department of Cataract, Pediatric Ophthalmology and Strabismus, Gomabai Netralaya and Research Centre, Neemuch, Madhya Pradesh, India

B. Gurnani, K. Kaur (eds.), *Atlas of Cornea*, https://doi.org/10.1007/978-981-96-0013-7_13

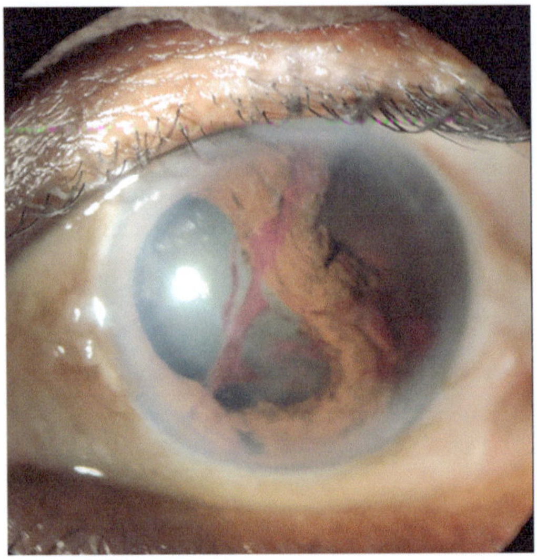

Slit lamp image in digital diffuse illumination of a 50-year-old male patient sustained a blunt trauma against the handle of the cycle bar in a road traffic accident in the left eye. The patient presented with corneal edema, anterior chamber was of moderate depth, irregular dilated pupil, and detached iris along 1 clock hour to 4 clock hours indicating iridodialysis, along with dispersed blood clots

13.2.2 Pseudophacocele

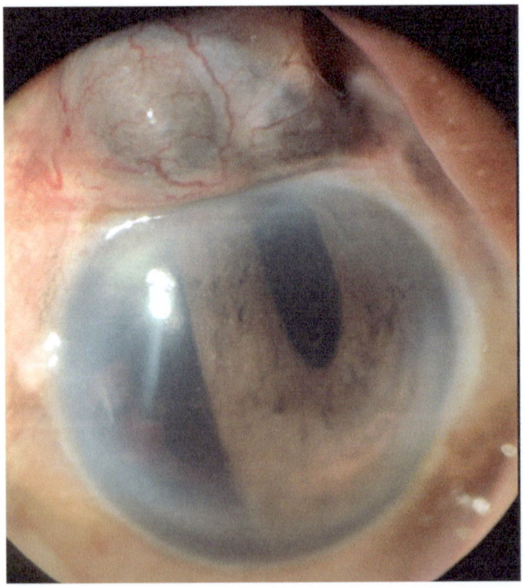

Slit lamp image on diffuse illumination in a 25-year-old male patient, who sustained cracker injury. He was a silent bystander during the incident. The patient had blunt trauma with large iridodialysis from 6 to 12 o' clock hours with a typical D-shaped pupil. The detached iris has prolapsed through the weak previous surgical SICS wound superiorly and covered by conjunctiva. Apart from the iritis, posterior intraocular lens is noted to be in place

13.2.3 Full-Thickness Corneal Laceration

13.2.3.1 Iris Prolapse with Eight-Ball Hyphema

Corneal perforation, resulting from trauma or corneal ulceration, presents with severe pain, decreased vision, and aqueous leakage. Prompt diagnosis through slit lamp examination and Seidel test is crucial. Treatment includes the application of a bandage contact lens, cyanoacrylate glue, or surgical repair with corneal grafting [3].

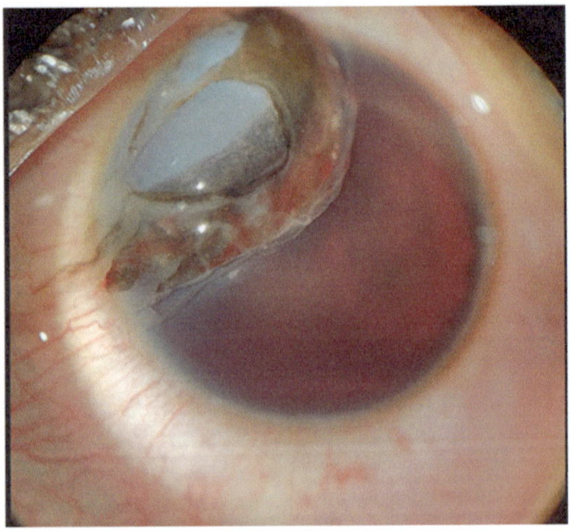

Diffuse illumination image shows a U-shaped full-thickness corneal laceration extending from 12 clock hours to 9 o' hours. The patient sustained the injury while in workplace, nailing the wall with a hammer. The corneal flap was detached and edematous with the prolapse of the vitreous and iris. The anterior chamber is completely filled with blood clots; there is no further view of the iris or lens details

13.2.4 Iris Prolapse with Corneal Edema

Limbal and scleral tears are traumatic disruptions at the limbus or sclera, respectively. These injuries can lead to significant structural and functional damage. Diagnosis involves detailed slit lamp examination and imaging. Treatment often requires surgical repair to restore ocular integrity and prevent further complications [4, 5].

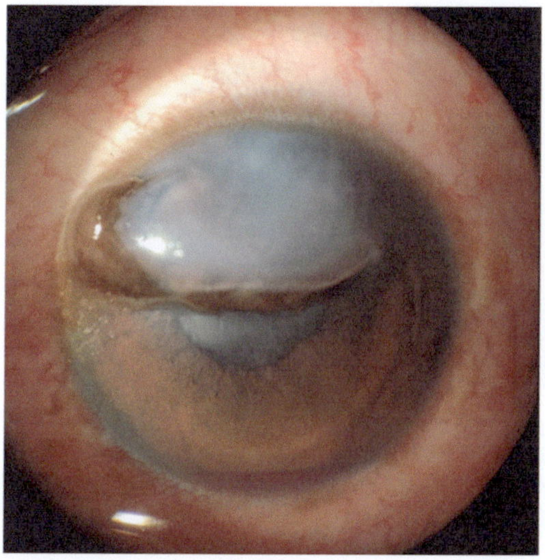

Slit lamp image of a 60-year-old female who sustained injury while feeding the calf by its horn. Full-thickness corneal laceration and edematous detached flap with iris prolapse. Rest of the cornea appears clear with trace hyphema in the anterior chamber. In addition, there is traumatic mydriasis due to sphincter tear noticed in the lower pupillary margin with traumatic cataract

13.2.5 Full-Thickness Limbal Corneal Tear with Iris Prolapse

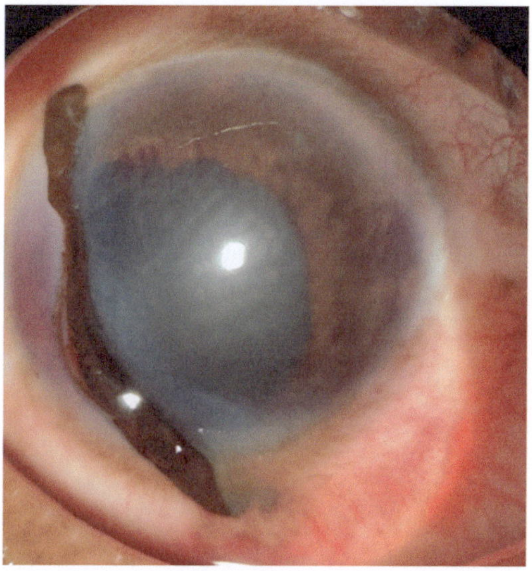

Diffuse slit lamp image of an open globe injury patient depicting a linear, vertical full-thickness limbal corneal tear extending from 11 clock hours to 7 o' clock hours limbus and into 1 mm sclera. The actual extent of the wound has to be explored before wound repair. The tear wound has prolapsed healthy iris tissue, anteriorly subluxated lens with intact lens capsule, and traumatic mydriasis

13.2.6 Small Iridodialysis with Exposed Ciliary Body

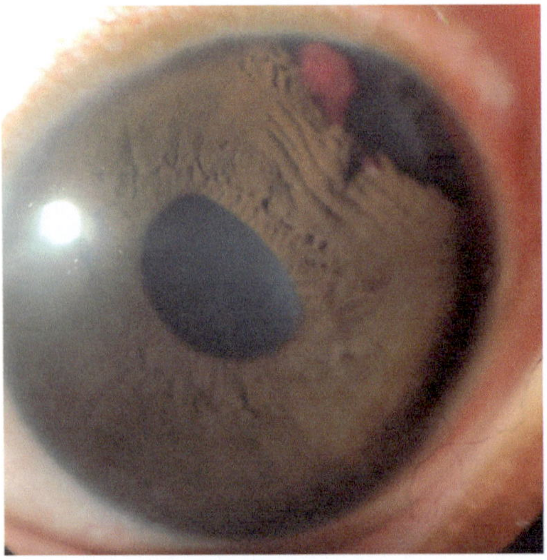

Corneal image of a 40-year-old female captured in a slit lamp under diffuse illumination. The image shows small iridodialysis with exposed ciliary body intact and blood clot. The iridodialysis extends from 12 clock hours to 2.30 o' clock hours. Mild corneal edema is seen with D-shaped pupil. The patient gave history of domestic violence by her husband with a wooden stick

13.2.7 Post-Corneal Tear Repair: Hyphema

Hyphema, the accumulation of blood in the anterior chamber, commonly results from blunt trauma. It presents with pain, photophobia, and blurred vision. Diagnosis is clinical, and management includes elevating the head, using cycloplegics, and monitoring intraocular pressure. Surgical intervention may be necessary for nonresolving or total hyphema [6].

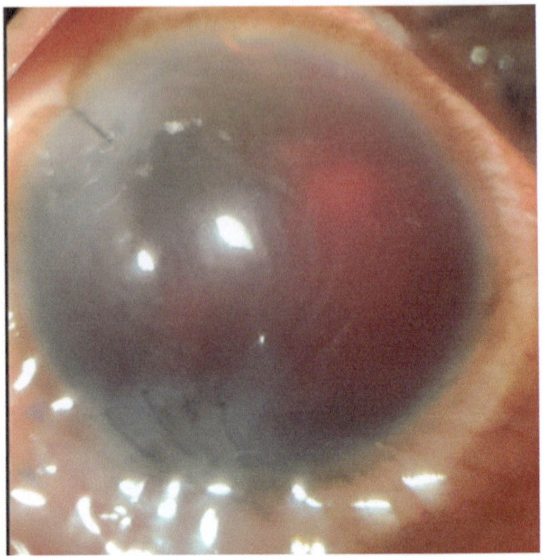

Image captured with diffuse illumination from a slit lamp in a smartphone camera. The image shows a sutured corneal tear inferiorly with 10-0 nylon sutures. A tight side port suture is noticed superiorly at 10 o' clock hours. Apart from the corneal edema, Descemet's membrane folds are noted due to the tight sutures. The anterior chamber shows rebleeding from iris following the wound repair

13.2.8 Corneal Abrasions

Corneal abrasions are superficial injuries to the corneal epithelium, presenting with pain, tearing, and photophobia. Diagnosis is confirmed by fluorescein staining. Treatment includes lubricating eye drops, topical antibiotics, and cycloplegics to promote healing and prevent infection [7].

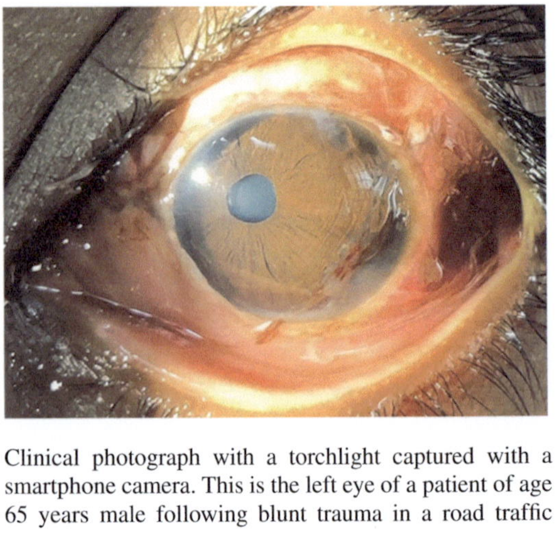

Clinical photograph with a torchlight captured with a smartphone camera. This is the left eye of a patient of age 65 years male following blunt trauma in a road traffic

accident. There is matting of eye lashes with epiphora due to corneal abrasions in the temporal paracentral zone of the cornea. Deep anterior chamber was noted with decentered pupil and partially torn iris along the nasal cornea

13.2.9 Toxic Keratopathy

Toxic keratopathy results from exposure to toxic substances such as chemicals or drugs. It presents with pain, redness, and epithelial defects. Diagnosis is based on history and clinical examination. Management involves discontinuing the offending agent and providing supportive care with lubricants and protective measures [8].

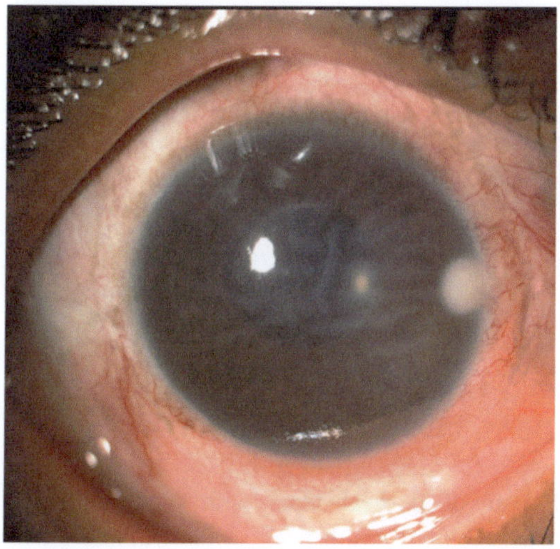

A 40-year-old male patient came with complaints of defective vision and photophobia for 2 days duration in the right eye. On diffuse illumination in a slit lamp, circumcorneal congestion was noted with diffuse Descemet's membrane folds from limbus to limbus, round, white full-thickness infiltrate noted at 3'o clock positive with the foreign body in situ. The anterior chamber was normal in depth with severe iritis, mid-dilated pupil, and a posterior chamber intraocular lens was present. On closer examination, the foreign body was noted to be the stinger from the bee. He was then diagnosed with toxic endothelial keratitis due to bee sting

13.2.10 Multiple Corneal Foreign Bodies

Corneal foreign bodies, either superficial or multiple, are common ocular injuries. They present with pain, foreign body sensation, and redness. Diagnosis involves slit lamp examination, and removal is typically performed under topical anesthesia using specialized instruments. Antibiotic prophylaxis is recommended post-removal [9, 10].

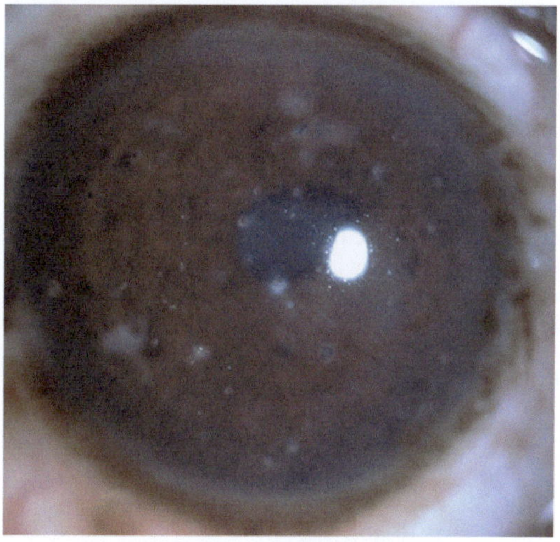

Picture seen with diffuse illumination in a slit lamp, captured with a mobile camera. Multiple foreign bodies embedded in the anterior stroma throughout the cornea. The size of foreign bodies varies from small to large with surrounding scarring. On close observation, the foreign bodies are the inert stones. The patient was having irritation and photophobia. The diagnosis made was accidental blast injury in a patient who was working in stone mines

13.2.11 Superficial Corneal Foreign Body

A superficial corneal foreign body is a common ocular injury where a foreign object, such as metal or organic material, adheres to the corneal surface. Symptoms include pain, tearing, and photophobia. Prompt removal using appropriate techniques, followed by antibiotic prophylaxis to prevent infection, is essential for optimal recovery [11].

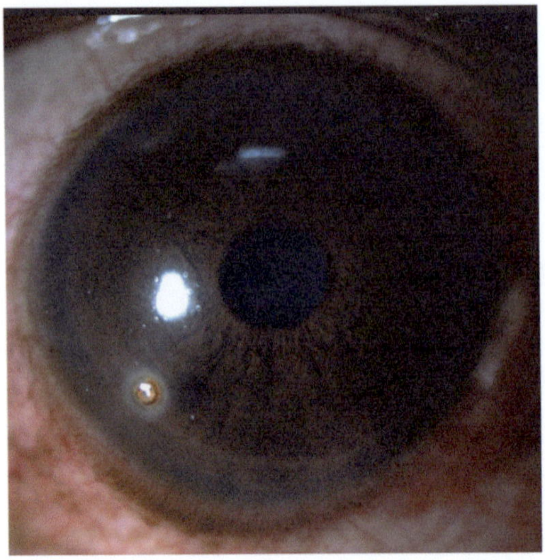

A 17-year-old male presented with severe foreign body sensation. Examination in a slit lamp, with diffuse illumination, revealed a circular, brownish elevated foreign body of size 1 mm, with surrounding scarring and minimal healing infiltrate. The foreign body is identified as an iron piece with a rust ring around it. This is the commonest forign body injury that occurs in welders. The protective eye wear prevents such occupational hazards

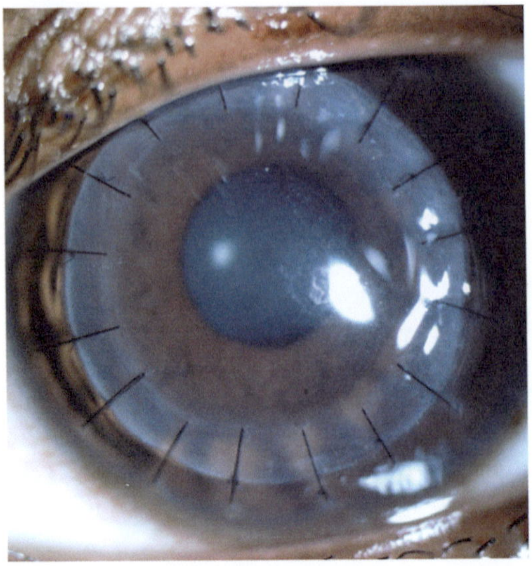

An 18-year-old female underwent deep anterior lamellar keratoplasty in the right eye for advanced keratoconus. The image above shows a clear graft of size 8 mm, circular secured with 16 interrupted 10–0 nylon sutures. The intraoperative technique was Anwar's big bubble, type I. The anterior chamber is well formed, quiet with clear crystalline lens. The patient's vision improved postoperatively

13.2.12 Deep Anterior Lamellar Keratoplasty

13.2.12.1 Deep Anterior Lamellar Keratoplasty (DALK)

DALK is a surgical technique for treating deep corneal injuries without penetrating the endothelium. Indications include severe corneal scars or dystrophies. The procedure preserves the patient's endothelium, reducing the risk of rejection. Postoperative care includes topical steroids and antibiotics [12].

13.2.13 Post-Corneal Tear Repair with Iris Abscission

Repair of corneal tears with concurrent iris abscission can result from severe trauma. These cases require meticulous surgical intervention to restore structural integrity and functional outcomes. Postoperative management focuses on preventing infection and inflammation [13].

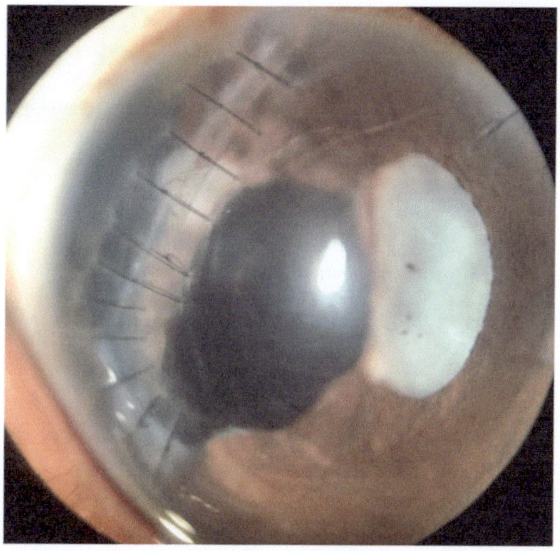

Slit lamp diffuse illumination image of a 12-year-old child after surgical repair of a penetrating injury to the eye. The clinical image shows a well-opposed corneal tear maintaining the obliquity of the cornea and irregular pupil due to iris abscission. The sutures are taken such that the contour of the cornea is maintained, reducing astigmatism in this case. The lens status is aphakic with the presence of partially absorbed cataract in the periphery

13.2.14 Entrapped Cracker Particles and After-Flap Wash

Thermal injuries to the eye result from exposure to high temperatures or radiation, presenting with pain, redness, and potential epithelial defects. Diagnosis is clinical, and management involves cooling the eye, using lubricants, and preventing infection [14].

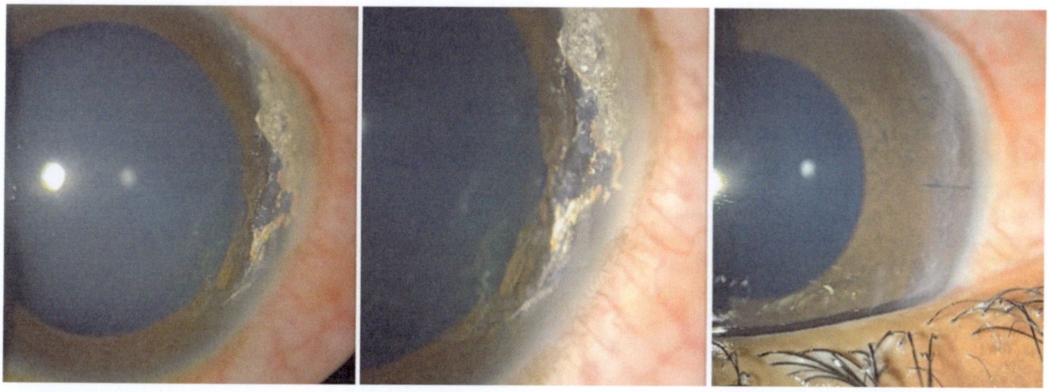

Slit lamp image of a 15-year-old boy who presented to our clinic after a firecracker burst near his eye 3 days back. Clinical examination revealed conjunctival congestion and a temporal lamellar corneal laceration from 2 to 4 o'clock at the limbus, with intralamellar silver deposition suggestive of cracker particles. As cracker particles contain sulfur and nitrate compounds but can also be inert due to the thermal reaction, reports of ocular toxicity due to these materials are reported. This boy was surgically treated with lamellar flap wash to remove the particles, and the wound was secured with 10-0 nylon sutures

13.2.15 Toxic Endotheliitis

Toxic endotheliitis is an inflammatory reaction of the corneal endothelium to toxic agents, leading to endothelial cell damage and corneal edema. Diagnosis involves clinical examination and exclusion of infectious causes. Management includes removing the offending agent and using anti-inflammatory medications [15].

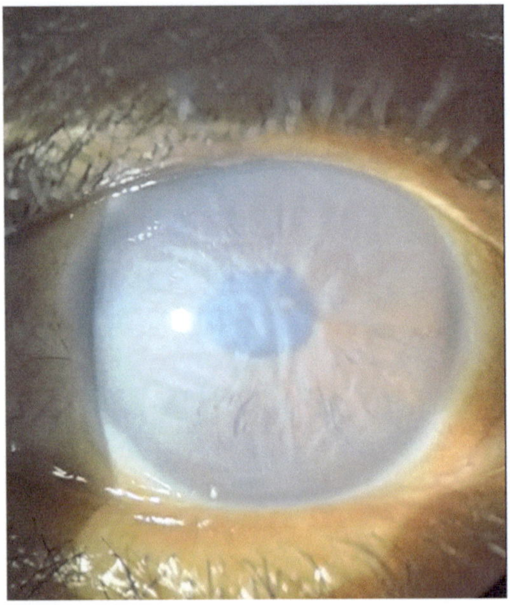

Slit lamp image of a 43-year-old female who presented with pain and defective vision of 1 day duration following exposure to some plant during farming. Clinical exam revealed conjunctival congestion, diffuse wavy lines over the posterior cornea with increased corneal thickness suggestive of Descemet membrane folds and stromal edema. The pupil was round, and well-centered anterior chamber reaction and lens details could not be made out. The acute presentation and the clinical picture point to toxic endotheliitis most commonly secondary to madar juice exposure in South India. Such a clinical picture should be differentiated from other causes of endothelial decompensation like pseudophakic bullous keratopathy, Fuchs corneal dystrophy, etc.

13.2.16 Open Globe Injury with Edematous Flap

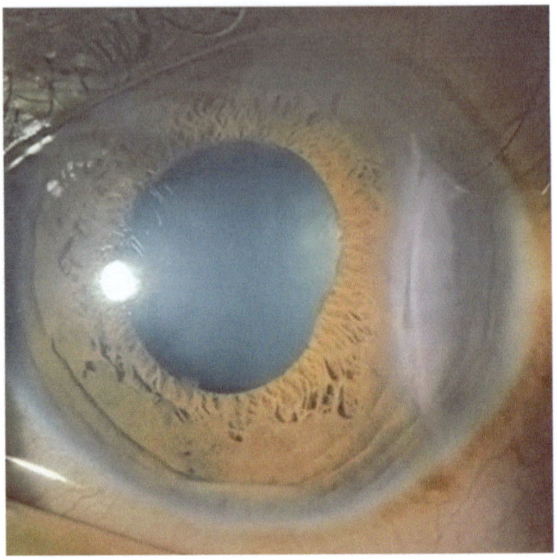

Slit lamp biomicroscopy image of a 15-year-old boy following a history of injury to the eye with a knife. The image shows a linear full-thickness penetrating corneal tear with clean, edematous edges. The tear is from 2 to 4 o'clock at the paracentral cornea, with an oblique orientation like a shelved wound, and traumatic mydriasis of the pupil can also be seen. Underlying lens is clear

13.2.17 Self-Sealed Corneal Tear

A self-sealed corneal tear is a partial-thickness laceration of the cornea that closes spontaneously without the need for surgical intervention. Management typically includes monitoring for infection, use of prophylactic antibiotics, and frequent follow-up to ensure proper healing and to prevent complications such as infection or corneal scarring [16].

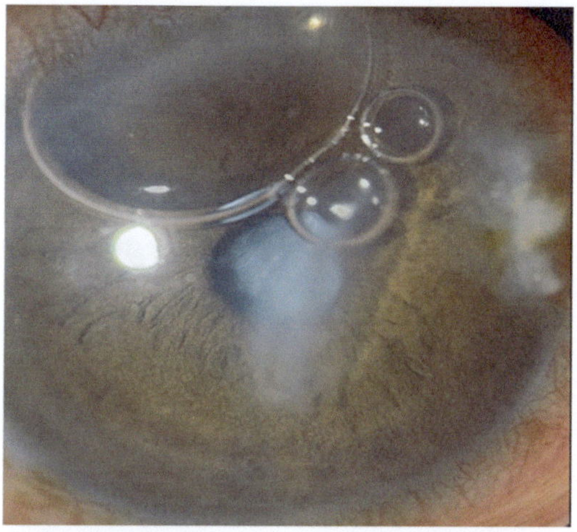

Self-sealed tear presented to us late with trapped AB. This is a slit lamp image of a 45-year-old male who presented to us with complaints of defective vision following a stick injury to the eye. Vision was reduced to hand movement, and clinical examination revealed a self-sealed linear corneal tear in the visual axis measuring 3 × 0.5 mm, oblique orientation, and a shallow anterior chamber. AC revealed the presence of entrapped air bubbles and traumatic cataractous lens. The force of the stick could have pushed atmospheric air inside the eye, and the oblique nature of the laceration could have caused it to be entrapped in the AC

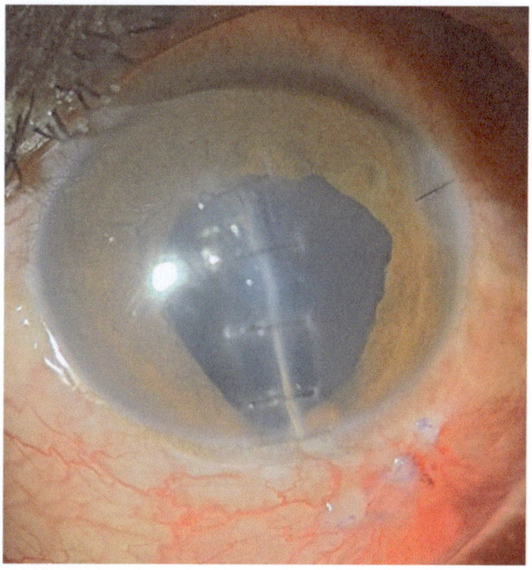

Fig. 13.1 Slit lamp image of a 50-year-old female, taken on a smartphone camera, revealing a postoperative clinical image of a well-opposed linear corneal tear involving the visual axis. The tear is opposed with five 10-0 nylon sutures, aphakia due to traumatic cataract extraction, and the underlying posterior capsule appears intact. The scleral extent of the wound has been explored intraoperatively at the 6 o'clock limbus; the conjunctival overlying it is apposed with a 8-0 Vicryl suture; anterior chamber is well formed with a side port suture at 2 o'clock limbus

13.2.18 Open Globe Injury Repair with Aphakia

See Fig. 13.1.

13.2.19 Traumatic Intralenticular Abscess with Hypopyon

An intralenticular abscess is a rare ocular condition characterized by the presence of a localized infection within the lens. It can occur following penetrating trauma or intraocular surgery and presents with symptoms such as pain, decreased vision, and inflammation. Treatment typically involves prompt surgical intervention to remove the abscess and prevent further complications [17].

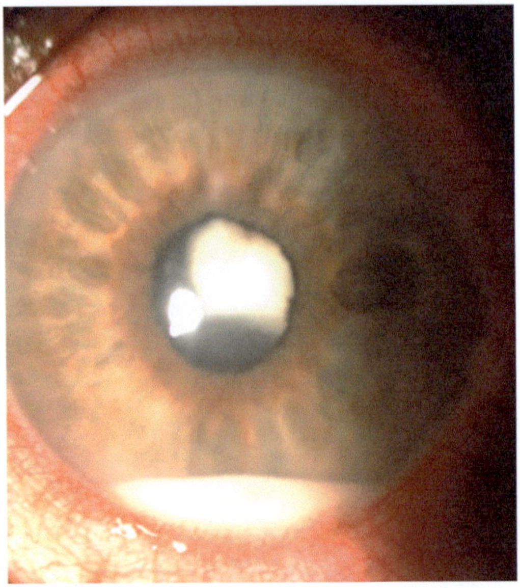

Slit lamp microscopy image of a 45-year-old male patient who presented with pain and sudden onset of defective vision. Clinical picture revealed the presence of hypopyon of 1 mm in the anterior chamber, iritis with circumcorneal congestion. A fluffy white-yellowish, localized opacification of the lens was seen at the pupillary area suggestive of a lenticular abscess. Detailed history of trauma, systemic status for immunosuppression (diabetes mellitus) and sign of penetrating injury should be carefully looked for in such cases. Intraoperatively, efforts should be made to localize any embedded lenticular foreign body during cataract extraction under topical antibiotic coverage

13.2.20 Traumatic Cataract

Traumatic cataract occurs due to direct or indirect ocular trauma, leading to lens opacity and visual impairment. Management often requires surgical intervention to remove the damaged lens and implant an intraocular lens to restore vision [18, 19].

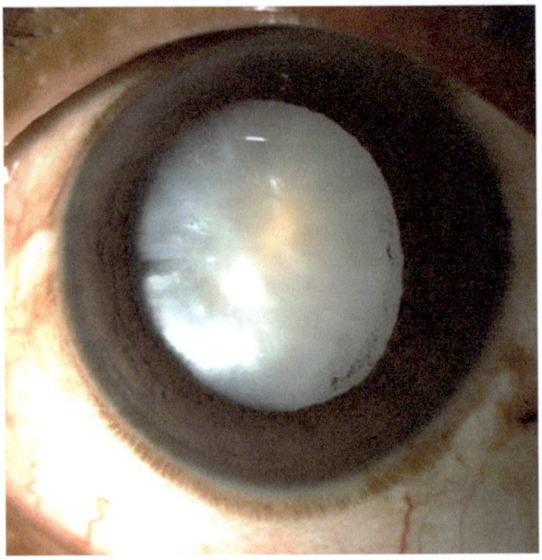

Clinical image of a 38-year-old patient who presented 1 month after suffering from a penetrating injury by a thorn. The anterior chamber is well formed, pupil is pharmacologically dilated, and there is a presence of intumescent, traumatic cataract with the anterior lens capsule breach at the 9 o'clock pupillary edge. The corneal scar as a result of the injury is obscured due to the white cataract

13.2.21 Open Globe Injury Repair with Traumatic Cataract

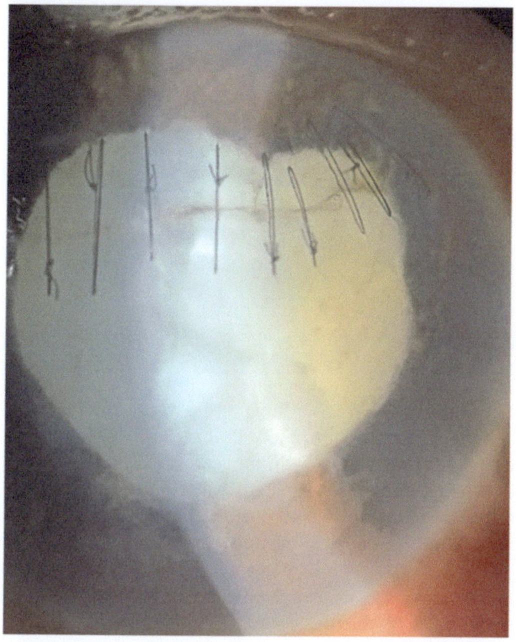

Slit image taken from a smartphone on a slit lamp biomicroscope. A linear full thickness corneal laceration is apposed with 10-0 nylon sutures with few iris pigments at the wound interface. The anterior chamber is shallow due to the anterior lens capsular breach causing traumatic, intumescent cataract, with the lens material seen floating in the anterior chamber, iritis, and an acutely inflamed eye

13.2.22 Fishhook Injury

Fishhook injuries to the eye are rare but can cause significant ocular trauma, including corneal lacerations and intraocular penetration. Prompt and careful removal of the fishhook, along with appropriate surgical repair and antibiotic therapy, is essential to prevent infection and preserve vision [20].

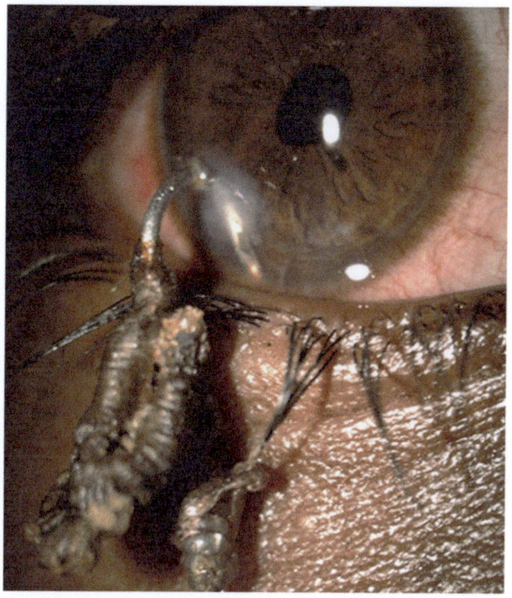

Slit lamp image taken under diffuse illumination of a 11-year-old young boy following a history of injury while fishing with his father. A full-thickness penetrating injury of the cornea is seen with a fishhook attached to the site of the wound at the 7 o'clock periphery, entangled with iris tissue. The pupil is round with no incarceration at the wound, and lens is clear. The patient was unable to close his eyes and was taken for emergency surgery to remove the intraocular foreign body under general anesthesia

13.3 LASIK Flap

13.3.1 Traumatic Dislocation

Dislocation of the LASIK flap due to trauma presents with pain, blurred vision, and flap displacement. Immediate repositioning of the flap and use of a bandage contact lens are critical for optimal recovery [21].

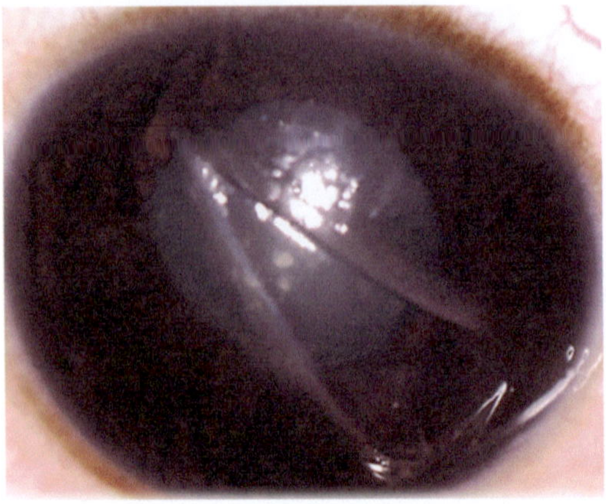

Diffuse slit lamp microscopy image of a 30-year-old male, with a past history of refractive procedure (LASIK laser in situ keratomileusis) and who suffered from defective vision after a cardiac surgery. He presented 4 months later with a visual acuity of 6/60 and a clinical picture revealing a central triangular defect with underlying hazy and epithelial ingrowth suggestive of traumatic dislocation of the LASIK flap due to some intraoperative manipulation. The flap shows two macrofolds, fine microfolds, and edematous edges with epithelial ingrowth. He underwent successful repositioning of the flap along with flap wash; the flap was secured with 10-0 nylon sutures to the underlying stromal bed

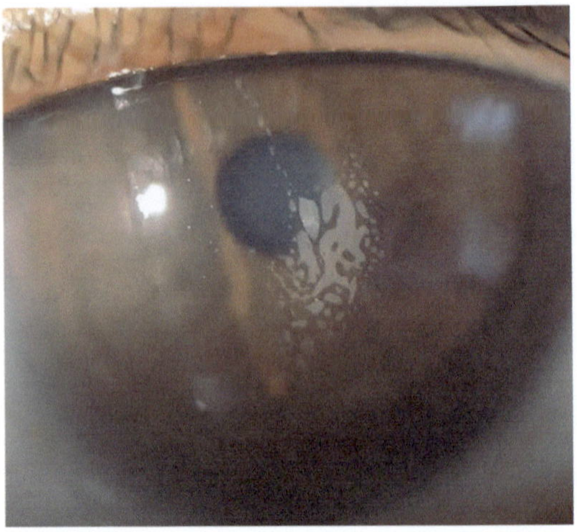

Slit lamp biomicroscopy image of a young female who underwent LASIK procedure 2 years back and suffered from accidental injury with the nail of her son 2 months back. She presented 2 months after injury during the Covid-19 pandemic with this clinical picture. The LASIK flap has folded on itself causing a macrofold from 6 to 11 o'clock, with the underlying presence of white plaque measuring 4 × 3 mm at the flap interface in the visual axis, suggestive of Grade 3 epithelial ingrowth (Jeffrey Machet's grading). The treatment for such a case includes surgical repositioning of the flap, with scraping of the ingrowth as well as the epithelium, along with a thorough wound wash to prevent recurrence

13.3.2 Epithelial Ingrowth

Epithelial ingrowth under a LASIK flap is a complication where epithelial cells migrate beneath the flap, leading to visual disturbances, flap melt, or irregular astigmatism. Treatment involves lifting the flap, removing the ingrown epithelium, and repositioning the flap to ensure proper healing and clear vision [22].

13.3.3 Stellate-Shaped Full-Thickness Corneal Tear

A stellate-shaped full-thickness corneal tear is a serious ocular injury characterized by star-like lacerations that penetrate the entire corneal thickness. Immediate surgical intervention is required to repair the tear, prevent infection, and restore corneal integrity and vision [23].

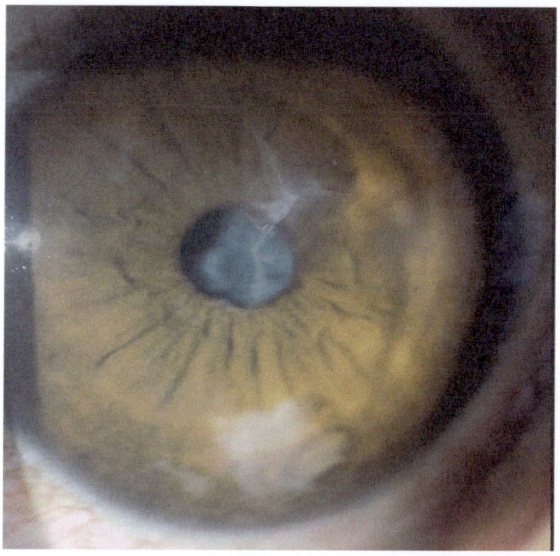

Stellate-shaped full-thickness corneal tear noted following a nail-and-hammer injury, seen with diffuse illumination captured with a slit lamp camera. The sphincter tear is noted in the inferior pupillary margin, and anterior lens capsular rupture is seen with nuclear matter in the anterior chamber

13.3.4 Corneal Scleral Tear with IOL Haptic Extrusion

A corneal scleral tear with IOL haptic extrusion is a severe ocular injury where a full-thickness laceration involves both the cornea and sclera, causing the intraocular lens (IOL) haptic to protrude through the wound. Immediate surgical repair is essential to reposition the IOL, close the wound, and prevent complications such as infection and vision loss [24].

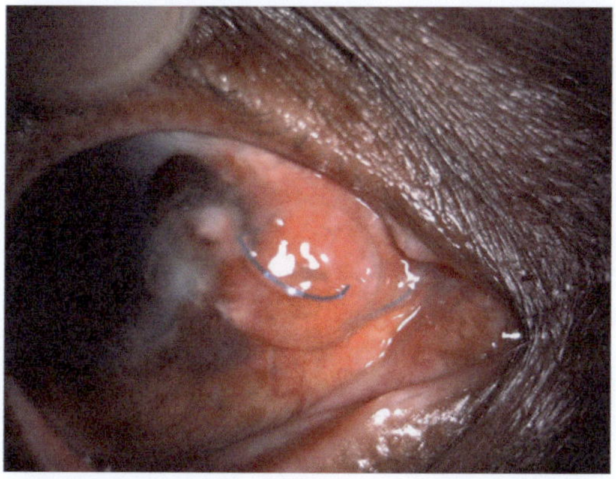

Diffuse illumination slit lamp image of an open globe injury patient depicting nasal corneoscleral tear with iris prolapse and extrusion of the IOL haptic from the wound site

13.3.5 Open Globe Injury with Pseudophacocele

Pseudophacocele refers to the herniation of intraocular lens (IOL) through a wound dehiscence or scleral defect after cataract surgery. This rare complication can result in visual disturbances and requires surgical intervention to reposition or replace the dislocated IOL [25].

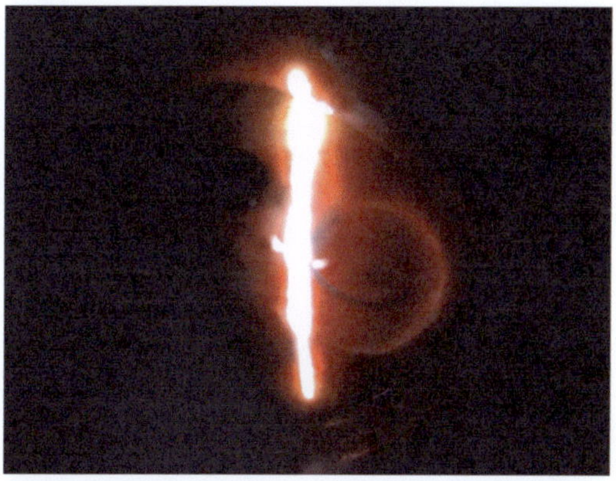

Diffuse illumination slit lamp image of an open globe injury patient depicting the extrusion of IOL from the bag subconjunctivally, suggestive of pseudophacocele

13.3.6 Post-Therapeutic Penetrating Keratoplasty

Therapeutic penetrating keratoplasty (TPK) is a surgical procedure performed to replace a diseased or damaged cornea with a donor cornea. Indications include severe corneal infections, corneal perforations, and nonhealing ulcers, aiming to restore corneal integrity, eliminate infection, and improve vision [26].

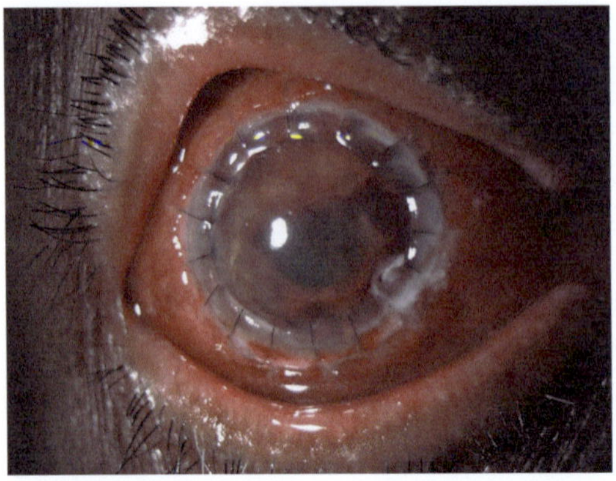

Diffuse illumination slit lamp image of a patient depicting a large clear corneal graft, well-opposed graft host junction, intact suture, well-formed anterior chamber, hyphema, and aphakia

13.3.7 Graft Edema

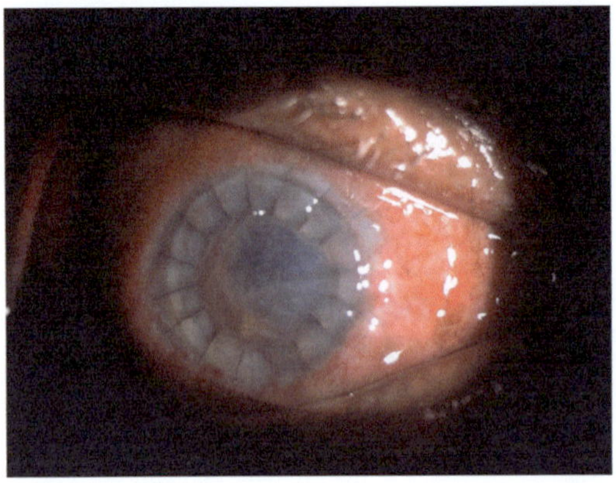

Diffuse illumination slit lamp image of a patient depicting a large clear corneal graft, well-opposed graft host junction, corneal stromal edema, intact suture, well-formed anterior chamber, and aphakia

13.3.8 Regraft for Graft Infection

Optical penetrating keratoplasty (PK) is a surgical procedure performed to replace a diseased or scarred cornea with a healthy donor cornea, aiming to restore vision. Indications include corneal dystrophies, scars, and keratoconus, where other treatments have failed to provide adequate visual improvement [27].

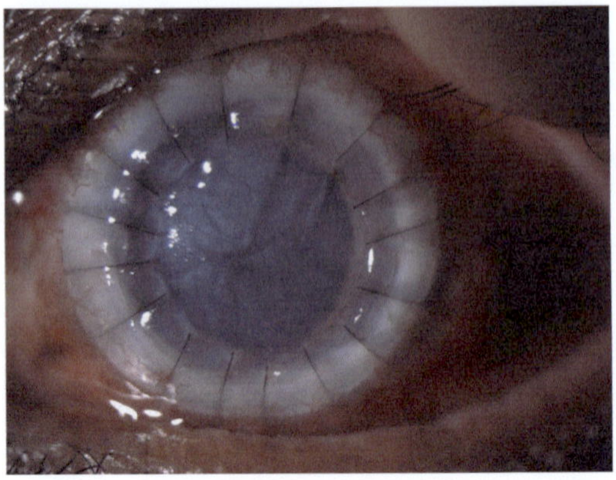

Diffuse illumination slit lamp image of a patient depicting a large corneal graft with stromal edema and well-opposed graft host junction with intact suture in a patient of graft infection post-optical penetrating keratoplasty

13.3.9 Failed Graft

A failed graft post-optical penetrating keratoplasty is characterized by the loss of clarity and function of the transplanted cornea, often due to immune rejection, infection, or endothelial cell loss. Management involves addressing the underlying cause, which may include medications or a repeat corneal transplantation to restore vision [28].

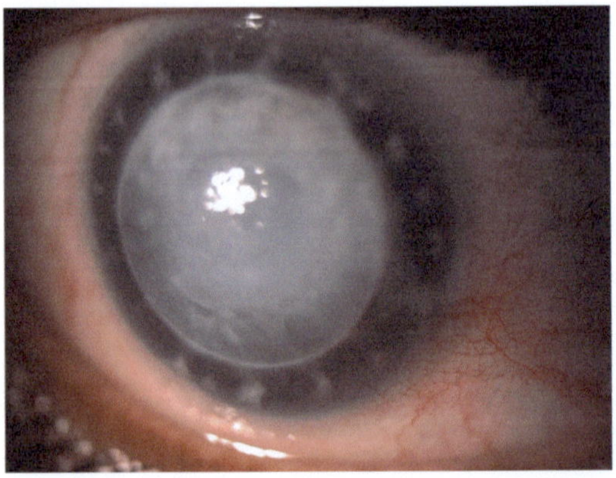

Diffuse illumination slit lamp image of a patient with total corneal opacification depicting failed corneal graft post-optical penetrating keratoplasty

13.3.10 Superficial Corneal Foreign Body with Infiltrate

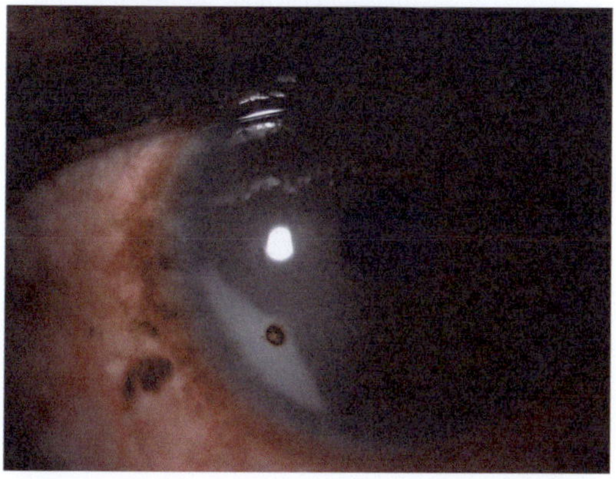

Diffuse illumination slit lamp image of a patient depicting superficial corneal foreign body with anterior stromal infiltration

13.3.11 Symblepharon Ring in a Patient Post-Chemical Injury

A symblepharon ring is used in patients post-chemical injury to prevent the formation of adhesions between the conjunctiva and the eyelid, known as symblepharon. This device helps maintain ocular surface anatomy, promote healing, and preserve eyelid mobility, crucial for visual rehabilitation and comfort [29].

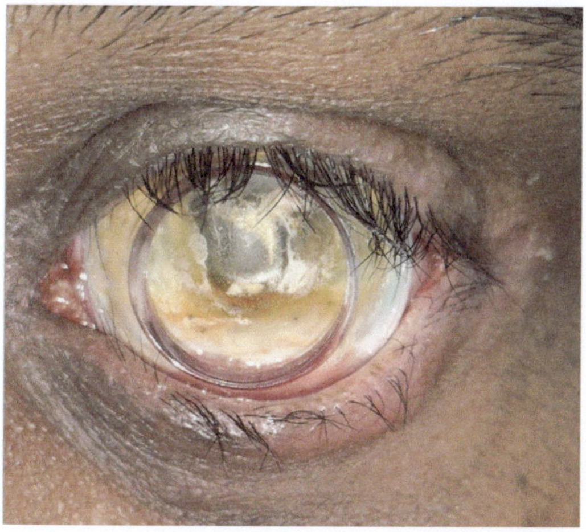

Digital image of a patient depicting the use of a symblepharon ring to stabilize the ocular surface and prevent symblepharon formation in a patient post-chemical injury

References

1. Sihota R, Tandon R. Parsons' diseases of the eye. 22nd ed. Amsterdam: Elsevier; 2015.
2. Vora GK, Demirel S, Wang H, Sheth S. Traumatic iridodialysis: clinical presentation and management. J Ophthalmol. 2016;2016:8235878.
3. Sharma N, Jain M, Sehra SV, Singh CP, Titiyal JS. Management of corneal perforation. Surv Ophthalmol. 2016;61(4):503–18.
4. O'Brien TP, Jeng BH, McDonald MB, Raizman MB. Limbal and scleral trauma. Int Ophthalmol Clin. 2017;57(2):69–84.
5. Vasan SK, Ramappa M, Murthy SI, Sangwan VS. Surgical repair of traumatic scleral lacerations. J Cataract Refract Surg. 2017;43(5):664–70.
6. Walton W, Von Hagen S, Grigorian R, Zarbin M. Management of traumatic hyphema. Surv Ophthalmol. 2016;61(3):297–303.
7. Chou R, Dana T, Bougatsos C. Diagnosis and management of corneal abrasions. Am Fam Physician. 2016;93(12):975–80.
8. Gupta PK, Tandon R, Gupta S, Sreenivas V, Vashist N, Satpathy G, et al. Toxic keratopathy: a review. Cont Lens Anterior Eye. 2016;39(4):350–8.
9. Cho BJ, Lee YN, Choi YS. Corneal foreign bodies: natural course and outcomes. Am J Ophthalmol. 2016;165:14–9.
10. Hoffman RS, Roufas A, Irvin LP. Management of corneal foreign bodies. Surv Ophthalmol. 2016;61(5):585–92.
11. Wagoner MD. Chemical injuries of the eye: current concepts in pathophysiology and therapy. Surv Ophthalmol. 1997;41(4):275–313.
12. Anwar M, Teichmann KD. Deep anterior lamellar keratoplasty: surgical techniques. Cornea. 2015;34(3):246–53.
13. Kook D, Funk RH, Ober MD, Sperling S, Rentsch FJ. Outcomes of corneal tear repair with iris abscission. Cornea. 2016;35(6):723–8.
14. Baradaran-Rafii A, Javadi MA, Rezaei Kanavi M, Jafarinasab MR, Rajabi MT. Management of thermal eye injuries. Surv Ophthalmol. 2015;60(4):322–38.
15. Huang MJ, Leu HB, Lin RS. Toxic endothelitis: diagnosis and management. J Cataract Refract Surg. 2017;43(8):1046–51.
16. McLeod SD, McLeod K, Eisen D, Brown SI. Nonsurgical management of corneal laceration. Ophthalmology. 1994;101(5):889–94.
17. Balamurugan S, Gurnani B, Kaur K, Gireesh P, Narayana S. Traumatic intralenticular abscess-what is so different? Indian J Radiol Imaging. 2020;30(1):92–4.
18. Chee SP, Ti SE, Sivakumar M, Tan DT. Traumatic cataract and intralenticular abscess management. Am J Ophthalmol. 2017;183:108–15.
19. Tiwari S, Ali MJ, Bansal R, Naik MN. Management of traumatic cataracts. Curr Opin Ophthalmol. 2016;27(1):32–8.

20. Hoffman RS, Capo H, Litoff D. Penetrating ocular fishhook injury. Am J Ophthalmol. 1990;110(6):676–7.
21. Stulting RD, Maloney RK, Mian SI. Traumatic dislocation of LASIK flaps: causes and management. J Refract Surg. 2016;32(6):372–80.
22. Leccisotti A. Epithelial ingrowth: incidence, diagnosis, and treatment. Clin Ophthalmol. 2008;2(3):673–5.
23. Smith PW, Stark WJ, Maumenee AE. Stellate corneal lacerations: surgical repair and visual results. Am J Ophthalmol. 1978;85(1):72–9.
24. Linebarger EJ, Hardten DR, Lindstrom RL. Management of dislocated intraocular lens. Curr Opin Ophthalmol. 2000;11(4):273–8.
25. Smith SD, Lee WB, Brubaker JD. Management of pseudophacocoele. J Cataract Refract Surg. 2017;43(11):1448–55.
26. Sukhija J, Jain AK. Therapeutic penetrating keratoplasty in infectious keratitis. Indian J Ophthalmol. 2005;53(3):169–70.
27. Bourne WM. Clinical indications for penetrating keratoplasty. Cornea. 1993;12(2):87–92.
28. Alldredge OC, Krachmer JH. Clinical types of corneal transplant rejection: their manifestations, frequency, preoperative correlates, and treatment. Arch Ophthalmol. 1981;99(4):599–604.
29. Donnenfeld ED, Holland EJ, Daya SM, Perry HD, Snyder RW, Stein RM. Management of the ocular surface in patients with corneal disease. J Cataract Refract Surg. 2004;30(9):1969–85.

Refractive Surgery

14

Arnav Singh Saroya, Soosan Jacob,
Bharat Gurnani, and Kirandeep Kaur

14.1 Introduction

Refractive surgery has revolutionized the correction of refractive errors, offering patients the possibility of reducing the dependence on glasses and contact lenses. The primary goal of these procedures is to reshape the cornea, thereby improving the eye's focusing ability. This chapter provides an overview of major refractive surgery techniques: photorefractive keratectomy (PRK), laser-assisted in situ keratomileusis (LASIK), small-incision lenticule extraction (SMILE), and radial keratotomy (RK).

14.2 Small-Incision Lenticule Extraction (SMILE)

14.2.1 Successful Docking

SMILE is a minimally invasive refractive surgery technique that involves creating a small incision in the cornea through which a lenticule of stromal tissue is extracted. This technique uses a femtosecond laser to cut the lenticule and the small incision, without creating a flap. SMILE offers several advantages, including the preservation of corneal biomechanics, a lower incidence of dry eye symptoms, and reduced postoperative discomfort [1, 2]. Studies have demonstrated that SMILE provides comparable visual and refractive outcomes to LASIK, with the added benefit of enhanced biomechanical stability [3, 4].

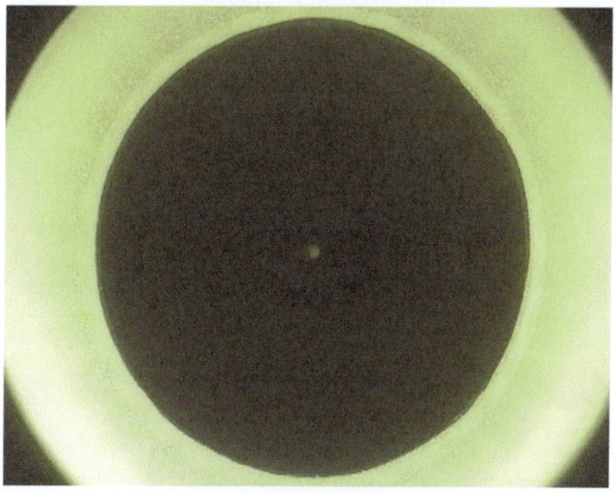

Diffuse illumination under the microscope image of a patient undergoing SMILE, depicting a central green pointer with successful docking

A. S. Saroya
Agarwal Eye Hospital, Cathedral Road, Chennai, India

S. Jacob (✉)
Cornea and Refractive Surgery, Agarwal Eye Hospital, Cathedral Road, Chennai, India

B. Gurnani
Department of Cataract, Cornea, Trauma, External Diseases, Ocular Surface and Refractive Services, Gomabai Netralaya and Research Centre, Neemuch, Madhya Pradesh, India

K. Kaur
Department of Cataract, Pediatric Ophthalmology and Strabismus, Gomabai Netralaya and Research Centre, Neemuch, Madhya Pradesh, India

B. Gurnani, K. Kaur (eds.), *Atlas of Cornea*, https://doi.org/10.1007/978-981-96-0013-7_14

14.2.2 Patient Centration

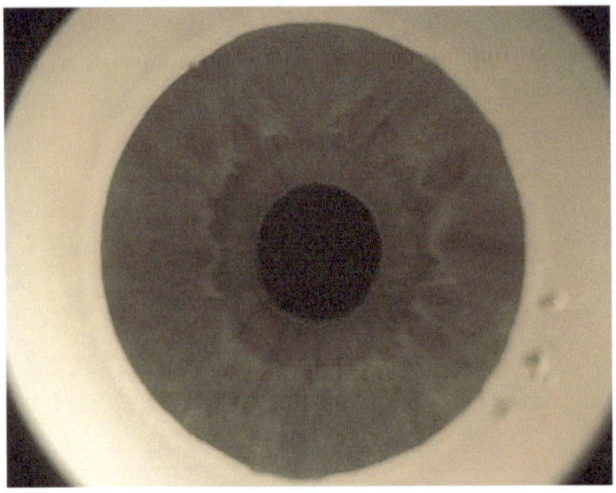

Infrared illumination under the microscope image of a patient undergoing SMILE to check for centration

14.2.3 Lenticule Cut

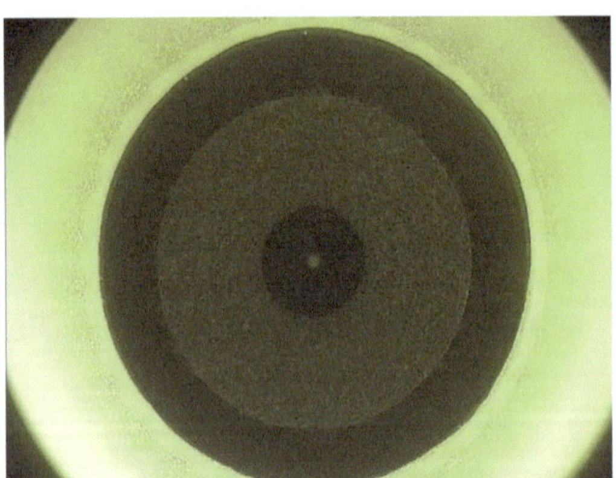

Diffuse illumination under the microscope image of a patient undergoing SMILE depicting lenticule cut from an outside-in manner

14.2.4 Lenticule Side Cut

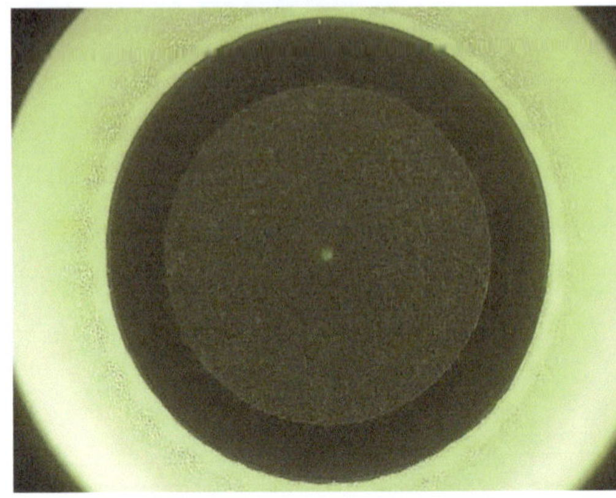

Diffuse illumination under the microscope image of a patient undergoing SMILE depicting lenticule side cut which is seen as a white reflex at the border of the lenticule

14.2.5 Cap Cut

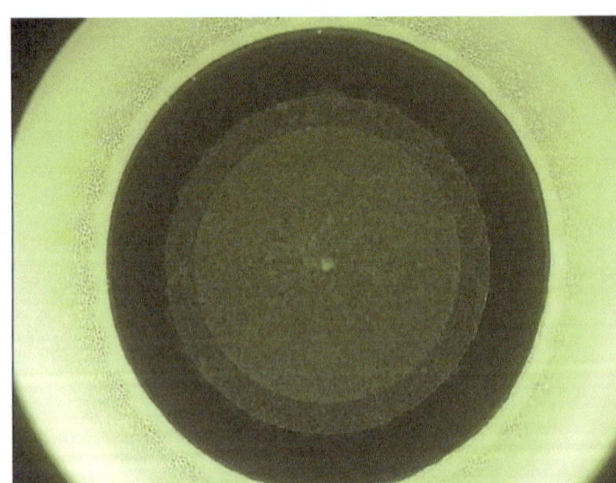

Diffuse illumination under the microscope image of a patient undergoing SMILE depicting cap cut from an inside-out manner

14.2.6 Cap Side Cut

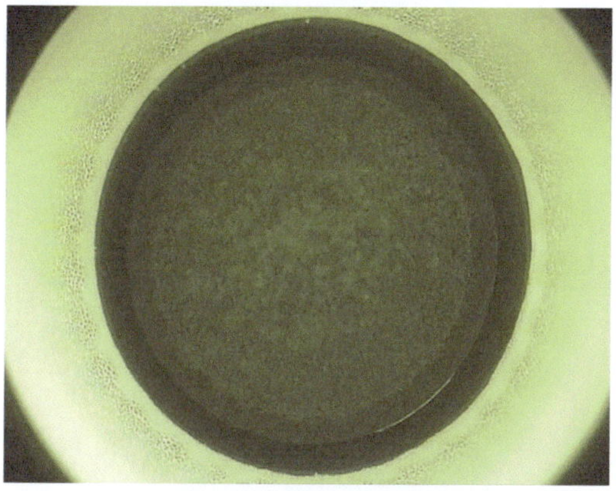

Diffuse illumination under the microscope image of a patient undergoing SMILE depicting cap side cut

14.2.7 Anterior and Posterior Laser Pass

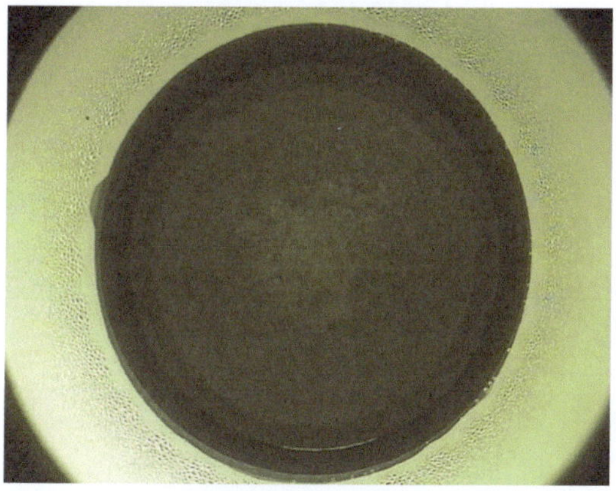

Diffuse illumination under the microscope image of a patient undergoing SMILE depicting normal anterior and posterior laser pass

14.2.8 Cap Side Cut Opening

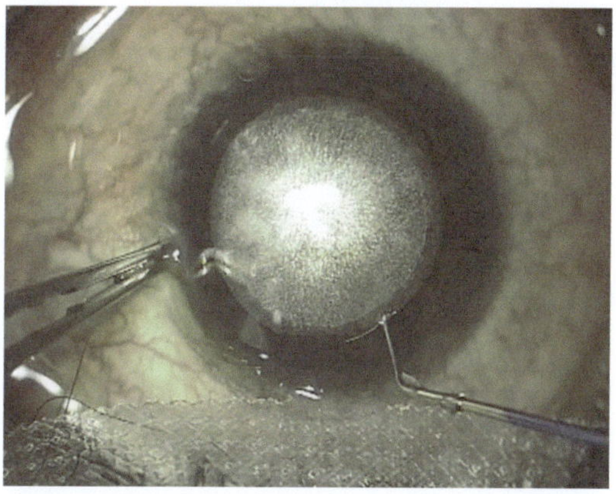

Diffuse illumination under the microscope image of a patient undergoing SMILE depicting opening of cap side cut

14.2.9 SMILE Incision

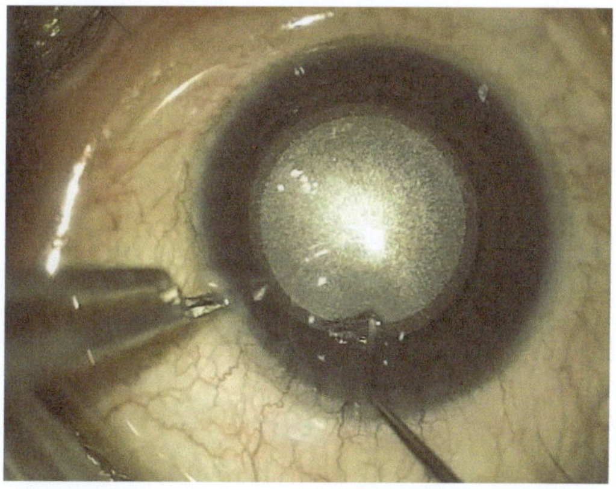

Diffuse illumination under the microscope image of a patient undergoing SMILE depicting 2 mm incision at 12 o' clock position

14.2.10 Anterior Dissection of Lenticule

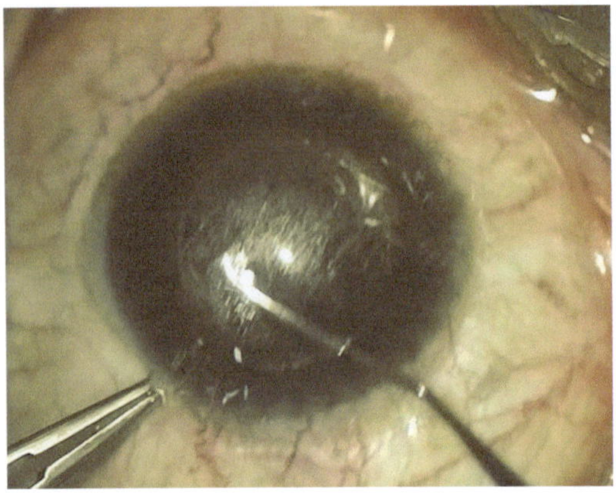

Diffuse illumination under the microscope image of a patient undergoing SMILE depicting anterior dissection of the lenticule

14.2.11 Anterior Pocket Dissection

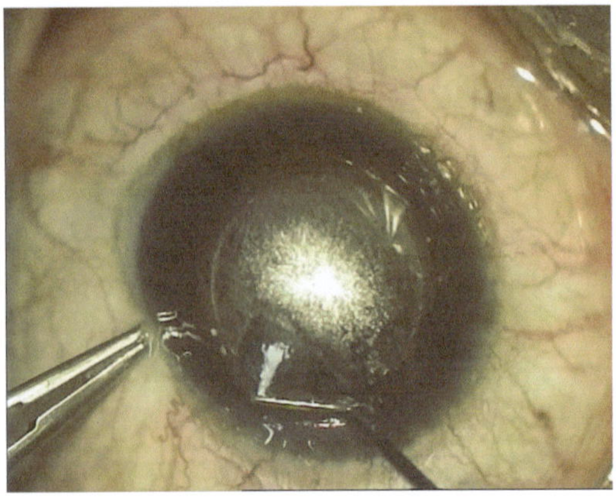

Diffuse illumination under the microscope image of a patient undergoing SMILE depicting complete dissection of the anterior pocket

14.2.12 Posterior Lenticule Dissection

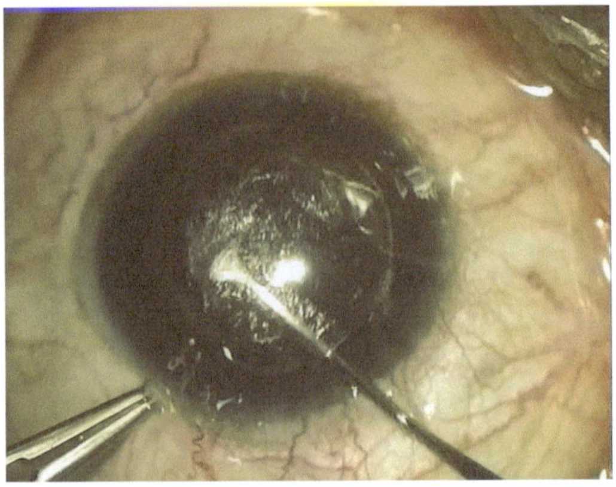

Diffuse illumination under the microscope image of a patient undergoing SMILE depicting posterior dissection of the lenticule

14.2.13 Complete Dissection of Posterior Pocket

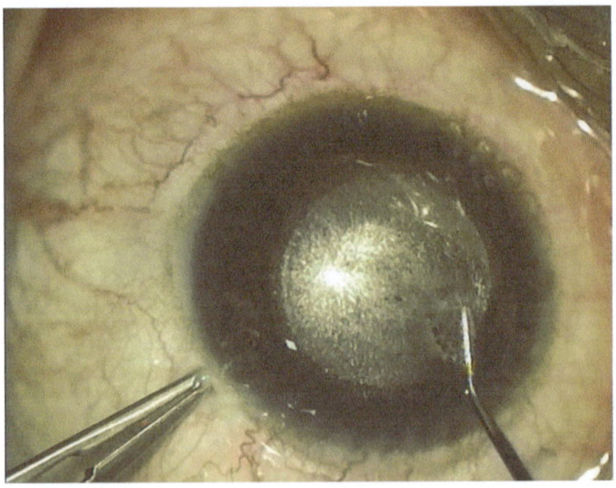

Diffuse illumination under the microscope image of a patient undergoing SMILE depicting complete dissection of the posterior pocket

14.2.14 Lenticule Extraction

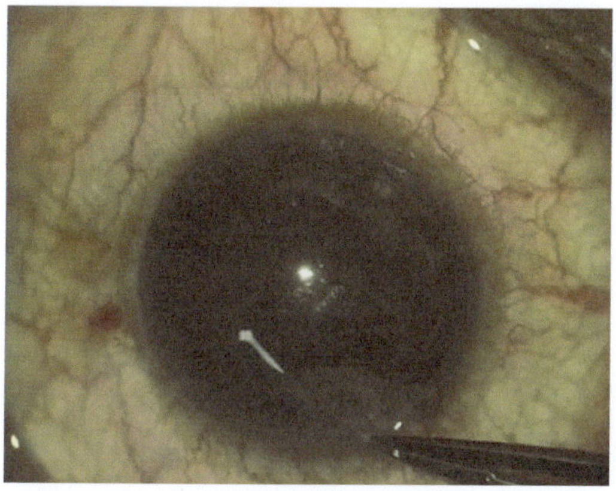

Diffuse illumination under the microscope image of a patient undergoing SMILE depicting lenticule extraction in toto

14.2.15 Cap Tear

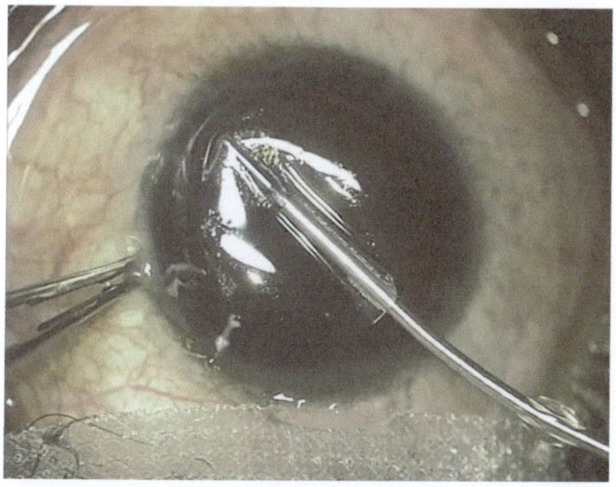

Diffuse illumination under the microscope image of a patient undergoing SMILE depicting cap tear

14.2.16 Dry Spot

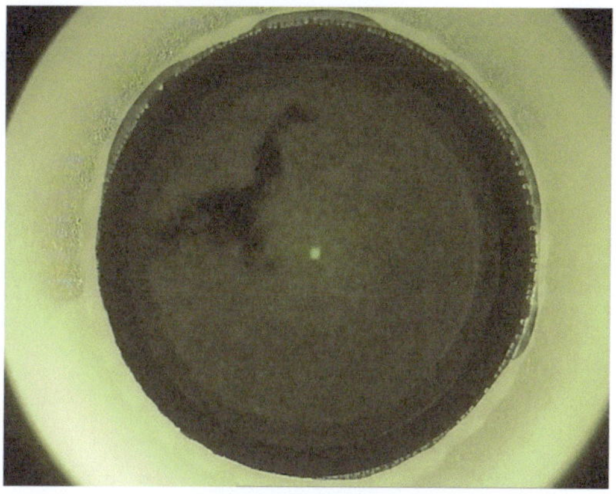

Diffuse illumination under the microscope image of a patient undergoing SMILE depicting dry spot

14.2.17 Excessive Dry Spots

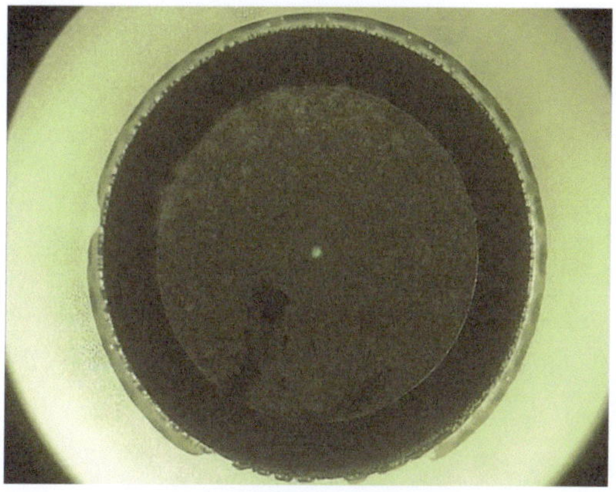

Diffuse illumination under the microscope image of a patient undergoing SMILE depicting excessive dry spots

14.2.18 Stuck Lenticule

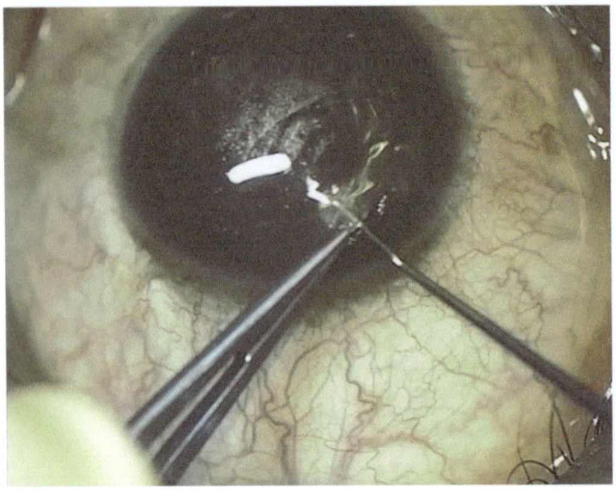

Diffuse illumination under the microscope image of a patient undergoing SMILE depicting stuck lenticule

14.2.19 Opaque Bubble Layer

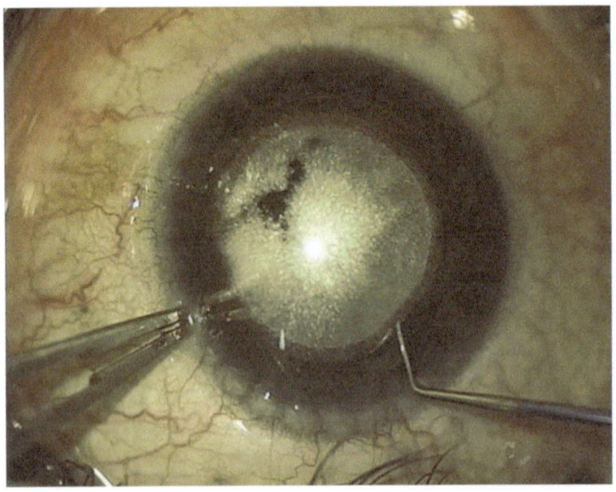

Diffuse illumination under the microscope image of a patient undergoing SMILE depicting opaque bubble layer

14.2.20 Suction Loss

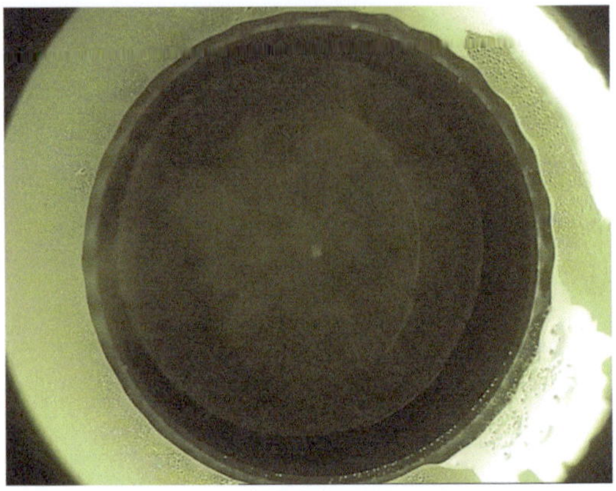

Diffuse illumination under the microscope image of a patient undergoing SMILE depicting partially created lenticule with suction loss

14.2.21 Impending Suction Loss

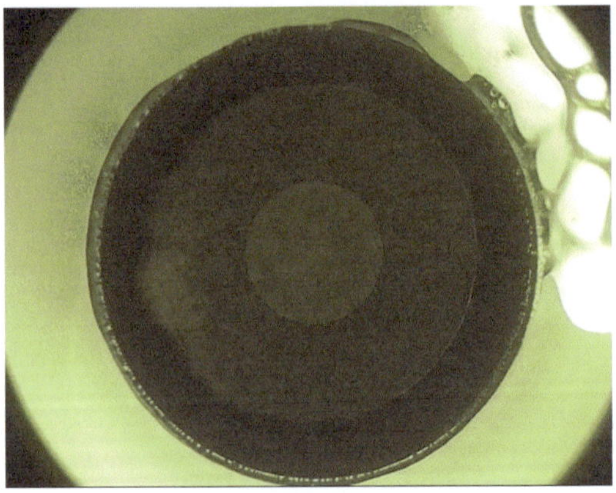

Diffuse illumination under the microscope image of a patient undergoing SMILE depicting impending suction loss. Notice the bubbles seeping under the SMILE cone interface

14.2.22 Lenticular Tag

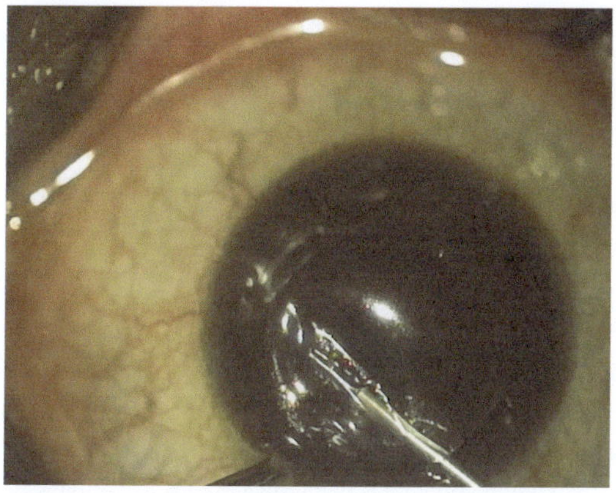

Diffuse illumination under the microscope image of a patient undergoing SMILE depicting lenticular tag

14.2.23 Black Spots: Interface Debris

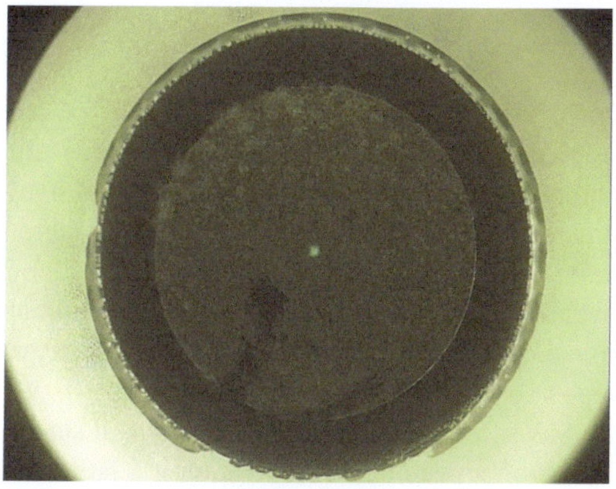

Diffuse illumination under the microscope image of a patient undergoing SMILE depicting black spots at sites of interface debris after laser

14.3 Photorefractive Keratectomy (PRK)

14.3.1 Laser Centration

PRK was the first successful laser vision correction procedure and remains a viable option, especially for patients with thin corneas or those at risk for trauma. The procedure involves the removal of the corneal epithelium followed by the reshaping of the stromal layer using an excimer laser. This results in a change in the cornea's refractive power. Although PRK requires a longer recovery period compared to LASIK, it offers comparable visual outcomes with a lower risk of flap-related complications [5, 6]. Advances in surface ablation techniques and postoperative care have further enhanced the safety and efficacy of PRK [7].

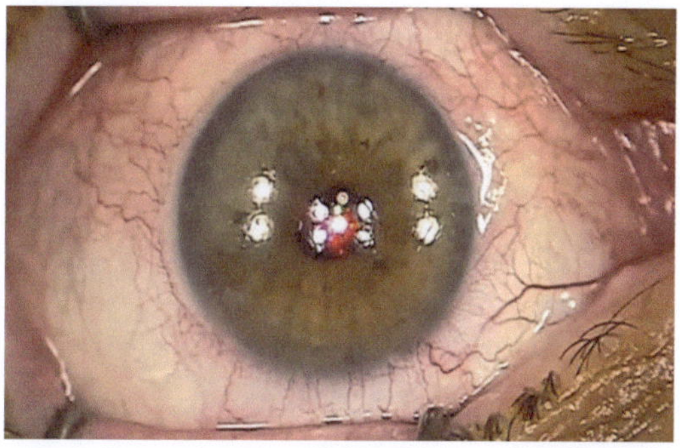

Diffuse illumination under the microscope image of a patient undergoing PRK depicting coincident red and green light with centration over the pupil

14.3.2 Epithelial Debridement

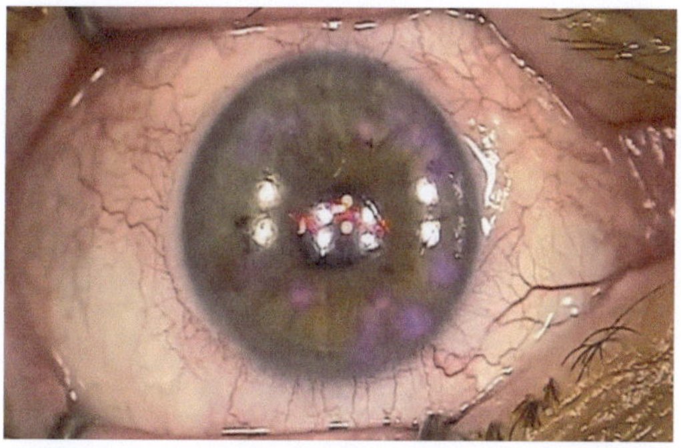

Diffuse illumination under the microscope image of a patient undergoing PRK depicting epithelial debridement using excimer laser

14.3.3 Stromal Ablation

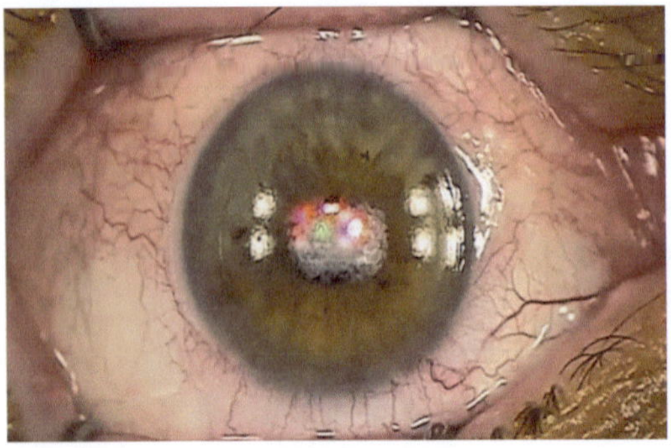

Diffuse illumination under the microscope image of a patient undergoing PRK depicting stromal ablation using streamlight PRK

14.3.4 Completed Stromal Ablation

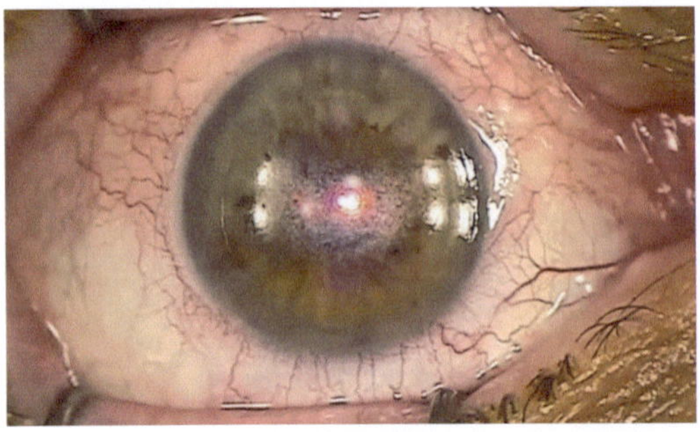

Diffuse illumination under the microscope image of a patient undergoing PRK depicting stromal ablation completed using laser

14.3.5 Mitomycin Application

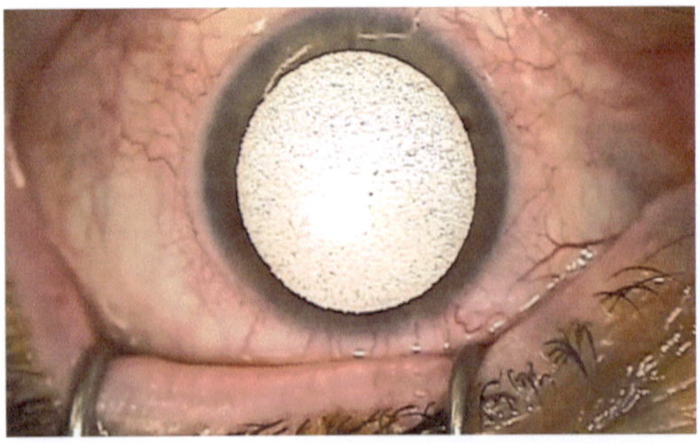

Diffuse illumination under the microscope image of a patient undergoing PRK depicting 0.02% mitomycin C-soaked pledget placed after ablation

14.3.6 Balance Salt Solution Wash

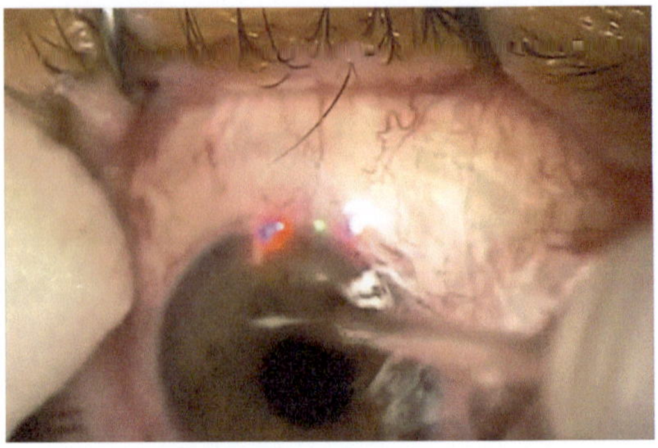

Diffuse illumination under the microscope image of a patient undergoing PRK depicting copious irrigation with BSS to wash off excess mitomycin C from the corneal surface

14.4 Laser In Situ Keratomileusis (LASIK)

14.4.1 Flat Cut

LASIK has become the most widely performed refractive surgery due to its rapid visual recovery and minimal discomfort. The procedure involves creating a thin corneal flap using either a microkeratome or a femtosecond laser, followed by excimer laser ablation of the underlying stromal tissue to reshape the cornea. The flap is then repositioned, adhering without sutures [8, 9]. LASIK offers excellent predictability and stability of refractive outcomes, making it a preferred choice for many patients. However, potential complications include flap dislocations, dry eye syndrome, and the risk of ectasia, particularly in patients with predisposing factors [10].

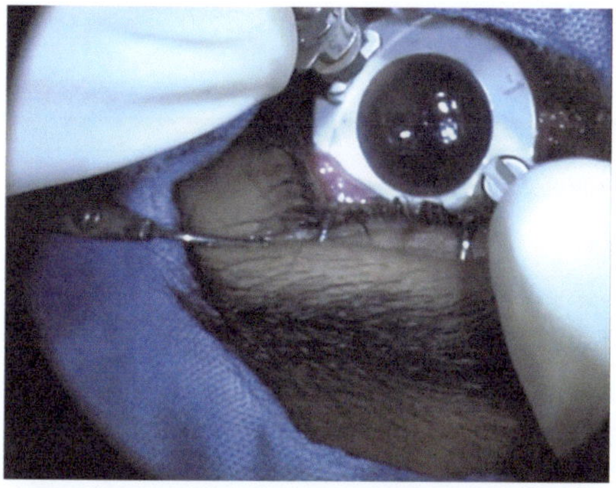

Diffuse illumination under the microscope image of a patient undergoing LASIK depicting flap cut with microkeratome application

14.4.2 Flap Lift

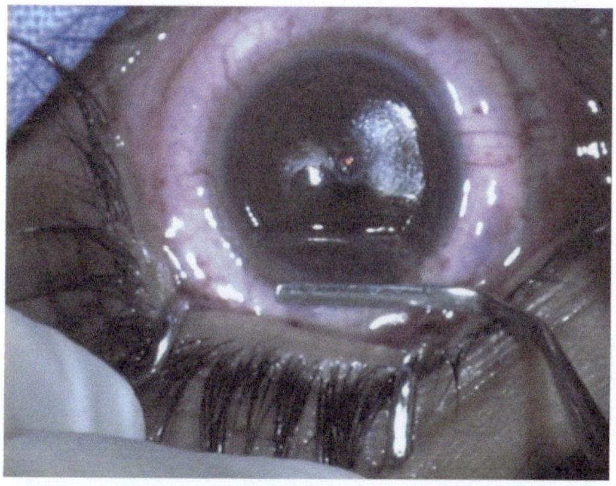

Diffuse illumination under the microscope image of a patient undergoing LASIK depicting successful flap lift with a spatula post-microkeratome cut

14.4.3 Stromal Ablation

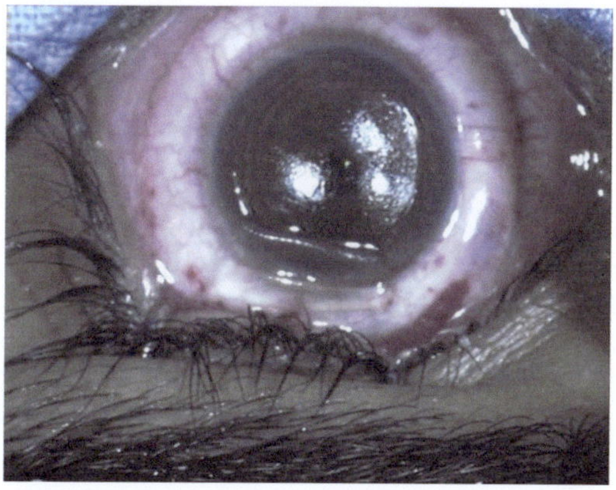

Diffuse illumination under the microscope image of a patient undergoing LASIK depicting excimer laser stromal ablation

14.4.4 Flap Wash

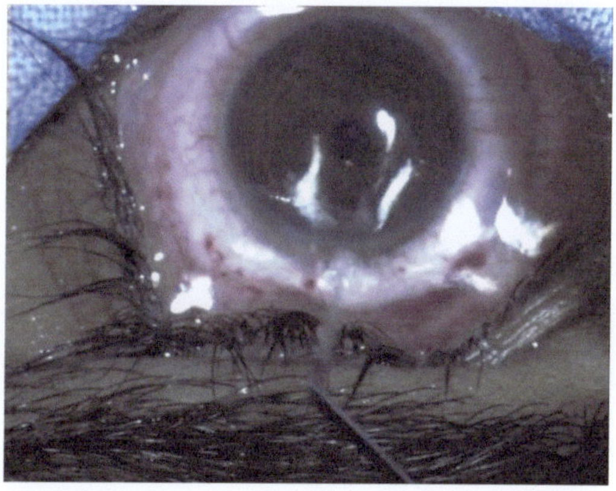

Diffuse illumination under the microscope image of a patient undergoing LASIK depicting flap wash

14.4.5 Flat Interface Wash

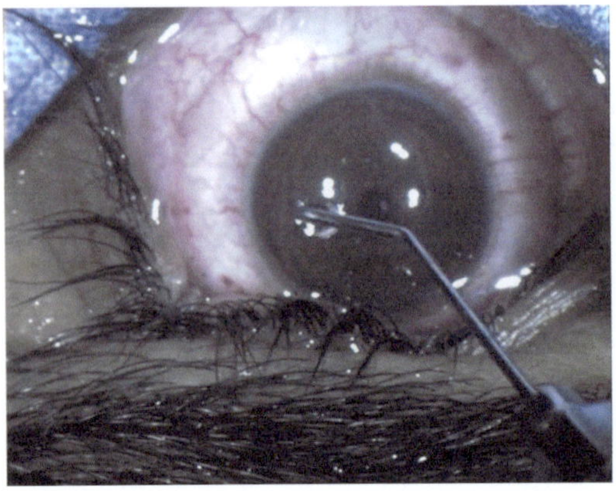

Diffuse illumination under the microscope image of a patient undergoing LASIK depicting flap interface wash

14.4.6 Decentered Flap

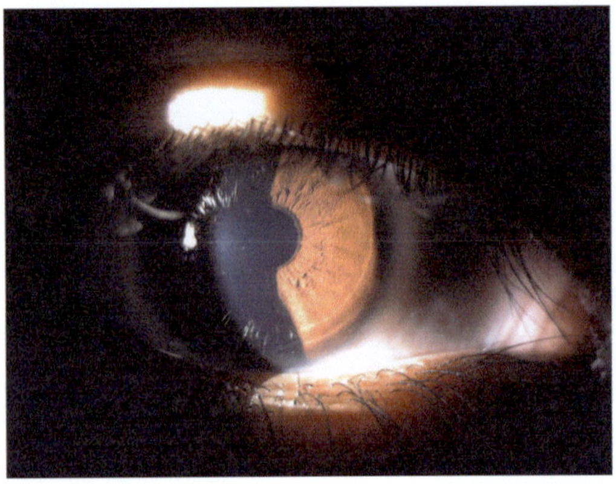

Slit lamp biomicroscope image of a patient depicting decentered LASIK flap

14.4.7 Traumatic Keratitis: Post-LASIK

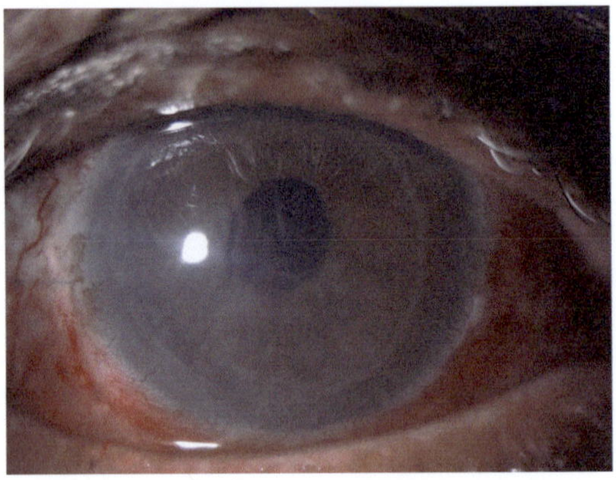

Diffuse illumination slit lamp image of a patient depicting traumatic keratopathy—post-LASIK

14.4.8 Post-LASIK: Infectious Keratitis

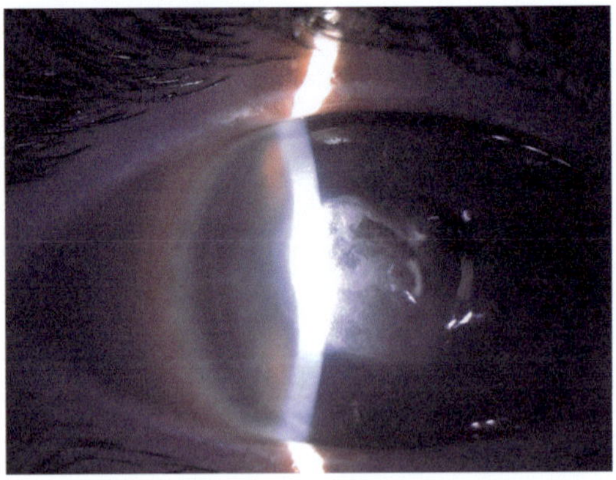

Slit illumination image of a patient depicting infectious keratitis post-LASIK

14.5 Radial Keratotomy

Radial keratotomy (RK) is one of the earlier refractive surgery techniques that involves making radial incisions in the cornea to flatten it and reduce myopia. Although largely replaced by laser-based procedures due to better precision and predictability, RK played a significant role in the evolution of refractive surgery. RK's long-term stability and the potential for progressive hyperopic shifts have been points of concern [11]. However, understanding its principles and outcomes has provided valuable insights into corneal biomechanics and the development of modern refractive techniques [12].

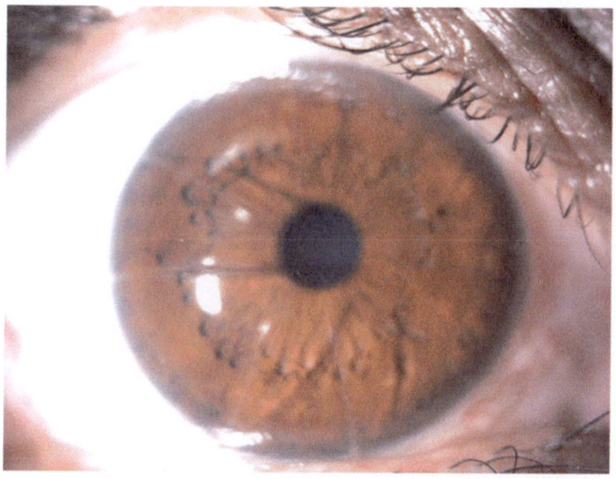

Diffuse illumination slit lamp image of a patient depicting post-radial keratotomy scars

References

1. Reinstein DZ, Archer TJ, Gobbe M. Small incision lenticule extraction (SMILE) history, fundamentals of a new refractive procedure and clinical outcomes. Eye Vis (Lond). 2014;1:7.
2. Blum M, Lauer AS, Kunert KS, Sekundo W. Outcomes of small incision lenticule extraction (SMILE) for myopia and myopic astigmatism: a review of the literature. Eye Vis (Lond). 2016;3:11.
3. Denoyer A, Landman E, Trinh L, Faure JF, Auclin F, Baudouin C. Dry eye disease after refractive surgery: comparative outcomes of small incision lenticule extraction versus LASIK. Ophthalmology. 2015;122(4):669–76.
4. Vestergaard A, Ivarsen A, Asp S, Hjortdal JO. Small-incision lenticule extraction for moderate to high myopia: predictability, safety, and patient satisfaction. J Cataract Refract Surg. 2016;42(2):200–7.
5. Waring GO, Reinstein DZ, Carr JD, Stulting RD, Thompson VM, Lynn MJ. Advances in corneal surface ablation techniques. Ophthalmology. 2016;123(5):890–8.
6. Fagerholm P. Photorefractive keratectomy: clinical results. J Cataract Refract Surg. 2015;41(3):457–71.
7. Shetty R, Kurian M, Ghosh A, Ramachandran S, Ashwini R, Kamat S, et al. Advances in photorefractive keratectomy techniques and outcomes. J Refract Surg. 2017;33(10):678–85.
8. Solomon KD, Fernndez de Castro LE, Sandoval HP, Biber JM, Groat B, Neff KD, et al. LASIK world literature review: quality of life and patient satisfaction. Ophthalmology. 2016;123(4):669–78.
9. Reinstein DZ, Archer TJ, Gobbe M. LASIK flap creation using the femtosecond laser: a prospective multicenter study. J Cataract Refract Surg. 2018;44(3):351–7.
10. Randleman JB, Woodward M, Lynn MJ, Stulting RD. Risk factors for ectasia after LASIK. Ophthalmology. 2015;122(8):1768–75.
11. Waring GO, Lynn MJ, Culbertson W, Laibson PR, Lindstrom RL, McDonald MB, et al. Long-term visual outcomes and stability after radial keratotomy: a 20-year follow-up study. Ophthalmology. 2017;124(9):1281–8.
12. Roberts CJ. The cornea and wavefront customized corneal ablation. Am J Ophthalmol. 2015;140(4):539–47.

MIX
Papier aus verantwortungsvollen Quellen
Paper from responsible sources
FSC® C105338

If you have any concerns about our products,
you can contact us on
ProductSafety@springernature.com

In case Publisher is established outside the EU,
the EU authorized representative is:
Springer Nature Customer Service Center GmbH
Europaplatz 3, 69115 Heidelberg, Germany

Printed by Libri Plureos GmbH
in Hamburg, Germany